ANGELS AND ASCENSION

Integrate Celestial Energy for a Benevolent Life

channeled by **Rae Chandran**
with **Robert Mason Pollock**

Other Books by Rae Chandran with
Robert Mason Pollock

DNA of the Spirit, Volume 1

DNA of the Spirit, Volume 2

Dance of the Hands

Partner with Angels

Coming Soon

The Universal Codes of Creation

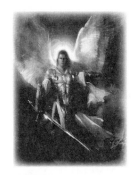
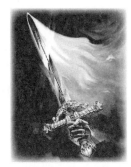
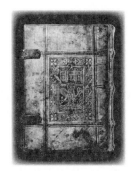

ANGELS AND ASCENSION

Integrate Celestial Energy for a Benevolent Life

channeled by **Rae Chandran**
with **Robert Mason Pollock**

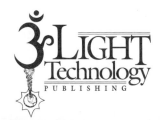

LIGHT Technology
PUBLISHING

For information about special discounts for bulk purchases, please contact Light Technology Publishing Special Sales at 1-800-450-0985 or publishing@LightTechnology.net.

Also available as an e-book from your favorite e-book distributor

ISBN-13: 978-1-62233-048-5
Published and printed in the United States of America by

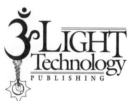

PO Box 3540
Flagstaff, AZ 86003
1-800-450-0985 or 928-526-1345
www.LightTechnology.com

Dedication

This book is dedicated to all the brothers and sisters on the path of self-discovery and self-love. May the wisdom from this book help you on your journeys.

This book is also dedicated to all the children of the world who are and will be the light carriers for changing humanity.

Acknowledgments

We extend our deepest appreciation and gratitude to precious Archangel Michael, who brought forth all the angels and other beings of light who contributed to this effort. We also extend our appreciation to these human angels: Cathy Clark, Fredaricka Yarrom, Mordechai Yashin, Deonna Phillips, Kevin Diamond, Christine St Clare, Amanda Sewell, Rebecca Cheung, Achutan Wong, and Yizhao Zhang.

Table of Contents

Spirit's Plan for These Times

Archangel Michael, Archangel Metatron, Archangel Gabriel, and Archangel Raphael

This is Archangel Michael. Once again, our gathering of lightbeings is a joyous and momentous occasion. It is recorded in your akash and Earth's akash. Always remember that every time you take a step to heal yourself, whether that is in the form of bringing forth a book or helping other people, you heal Mother Earth. We thank you for your participation, time, effort, and commitment to this work.

You are in an incredibly important time of change. There have been many naysayers regarding what is happening on Earth at this time, including some famous people who talk about mass extinction or one disaster after another. We foresee no major cataclysms. There will be changes, but Earth will not shift her poles, continents will not sink, and millions will not die. That is not Spirit's plan. We have worked hard to get this far. Do not believe the naysayers. Some have good intentions, and some have revealed wonderful understandings, but some people are caught in the matrix [mass consciousness]. Be aware of what you read, and have discernment.

There is a critical mass of people, and a shift is taking place. You will see more ugliness, and fearmongers will come forward. Look at the United States and what has happened in the past few weeks [the U.S. Supreme Court ruling on June 26, 2015, that recognizes same-sex marriages]. It is momentous and will go down in history as truly joyous, a day when liberation happened — the recognition of two beings in love, regardless of gender. This will be declared a day of great liberation in the years, decades, and centuries to come. Also, look at the removal of the

Confederate flag from government buildings. It took a long time for this to happen. Do you think this is a positive thing? We feel it is so. Good things are happening despite the atrocities taking place.

There will be a shift, and it will be a good shift. Bless all the naysayers and fearmongers, but develop your discernment.

✻   ✻   ✻

Healing Mother Earth

This is Archangel Metatron. We are overjoyed that the wisdom of angels is coming forth. This is the most appropriate way to bring about their understanding, for angels can completely transform your life and even your country.

You have such problems with pollution: seawater contamination, mining, oil spills, and excessive construction. All place great burdens on Mother Earth. There are angelic beings you can call on to heal these wounds. Some angels speak about what they can do with you to heal Mother Earth. There are certain criteria these angels examine in how you treat Mother Earth. For them, she is an extension of you, and when you treat her badly, you treat the bodies of other human beings badly as well. These angels also look at how you treat underprivileged people, animals, plants, and other creatures. But the main concern is how you treat your blessed Mother who gave you life.

✻   ✻   ✻

You Are a Celestial Being

We are Archangels Michael, Gabriel, Raphael, and Metatron. We hold energy and shower all of you with light and blessings for the journey you are undertaking in your life. We encourage you to work with archangels. You can visualize Metatron and Michael on your right side, Gabriel on your left side, and Raphael pouring light into you from all directions. You will see a massive expansion in everything you do. Call on the archangels. We can expand what you hold true in your heart and belief system. We encourage you to work with us.

You might say we are biased toward angels. Yes, we are biased, for we are angels. Your life can improve. Perhaps you have heard the expression, "Life is good, and it only gets better." You could say, "Life is good, and it only gets more celestial."

Hold this thought from now on: "I am a celestial being experiencing celestial energy from the angels, gods, goddesses, and All That Is. I am a celestial being. I am a quantum celestial being experiencing celestial energy every moment of my life."

The great teacher Lady Quan Yin instructs on celestial energy and how to integrate it. This is why she is called the master of the eleventh ray, which is for complete balance. Lady Quan Yin and Mother Mary are aspects of the same consciousness. She works with us angels. We encourage you to connect with Lady Quan Yin and with angels and archangels.

You can call us forth for any situation and in any part of your life where you need a boost. Just call on us. Whenever you feel you are in a bind, stand still and call us to be with you, inspire you, and guide you. We will be there in a second. We are here in service to you. Blessings.

❋　❋　❋

Physical Reactions to Shifting Planetary Energy

Greetings and great love to all of you. This is Archangel Metatron. We thank you for the opportunity to communicate with you, to bring you this interesting and wonderful information. Angels are available with all kinds of help. This must become part of your reality. Set your antenna to the angels, and communicate with them. All life's miracles happen with angelic presence. When you do this, you will see that you have an ever-present friend at your shoulder.

There has been a shift on this planet and in the human body. Many people are experiencing physical changes. This is sometimes uncomfortable. A part of your body might suddenly feel limp, and you have no energy. You might be taken to the hospital and for multiple tests only to be told, "You are fine." You might feel as if something is dramatically wrong and nobody is able to fix it. Many of you have had near-death experiences. Your bodies are shifting. Keep in mind that this could happen to you or someone you know, and it can be really frightening.

Work with Angels to Become a Light Warrior

All of you are incredible light warriors. A light warrior steps onto the battlefield. It is time for light warriors to be fully involved in everyday life: commerce, business, politics, engineering, medicine, science, and so on.

Spiritual activism must become an important part of your journey. Many say, "I am already doing two types of work. One is my personal work, and the other is working with Mother Earth." This is true, but you could also include the everyday world, for only when you influence the everyday world can you make positive changes. Perhaps you do not like your job. You don't like your company or coworkers, but please note that there is a purpose for being there: You are a light holder anchoring light.

If you request it, some of you will have the opportunity to connect with space brothers and sisters. Make this request in your meditations, "I ask for the grace of energies so that I can move forward and connect with my true family and benevolent brothers and sisters from outer realities and from all dimensions of time and space."

❋　❋　❋

This is Archangel Michael. Much support is available for humanity. Angelic support has always been available, but people did not know about it because they were looking for a tangible support system — something they could see, feel, or touch. In the new consciousness, you must learn to believe in the unseen. Know support is available if you focus.

The angels completely support every human soul on the planet as well as all animals, plants, and trees, but you must ask for this support system to be activated. We bring the understanding of angels so that you can work with them to find joy, peace, and freedom in your heart. We encourage you to speak with all your friends and family about the benefits of working with angels. Work with angels every day, and you will see the difference. Work with angels in every aspect of your life to see how this supports you.

There will be many transitions. There will be great fear among people, so talk with them about how to work with angels to bring peace to their hearts. Many people will be disturbed. They will see horror stories on the news and wonder whether the world has gone mad. You will see a distinction between the people who work with angelic energy and those who do not, and you will be able to lead them.

All of you have life contracts to be teachers of humanity through your regular jobs. Your life is your message. What message are you broadcasting every moment? Is it a message of empowerment, peace, joy, and freedom?

We would like to remind you once again that you are a soul having a physical incarnation. When people come into your life, be they coworkers, beggars on the street, or ticket collectors on a bus, there is a reason. Those people have come to receive a gift from you, and you are there to receive a gift from them.

What gift can you give? It is the memory that they are God. Hold this thought continually, especially in the first ninety seconds of meeting someone. Feel the energy flow through your physical body, and feel the other person's presence. Say to yourself, "I am the soul. I am my higher self." Then hold it. The people you encounter might remember who they are. This is the gift you give.

What is the gift you receive? It's an opportunity to express and exhibit this inner knowingness. The other person provides you with an opportunity to express this aspect of yourself. The exchange is perfect. Look for these opportunities every day and in every moment. The more you share, the more you give and the more you will receive. That is the secret of life. When you wake up in the morning, you can ask from your heart, "What is a gift I can share today? Is it a gift of knowingness? Today, I'd like to share the gift of compassion, kindness, or love," or it can be anything else. The more you do this, the more it becomes a part of your everyday life.

You are in a very precious time. Never forget that you can use this time to create a new reality for yourself. This has been a hard year with many ups and downs, but you are coming close to when you will be able to integrate higher energy and use it as part of your new reality. Focus on your abilities, feelings, and talents. Focus on your bigger dreams. You will be supported. Thank you, dear ones.

CHAPTER ONE

Enhance Your Senses and Vitality

Angel Barbiel, Archangel Michael, Angel El Varha, Angel Sanhriel,
Angel Vohumanah, and Angel Yahoel

This is Angel Barbiel. Most people experience life through their five senses, but these are only tools your mind uses to experience a desired reality. When you see something through your eyes, your mind sends them a command to see what it needs them to see, and it interprets it in the way it needs to interpret it. It is not the eyes that see. The mind sees and uses the eyes as tools. The same is true for what you hear. You hear what your mind wants you to listen to.

Clarify your Vision, Hearing, and Olfactory Senses

Bring your attention to both ears, and see two beautiful white and blue stars of David behind them emitting energy into them. This energy slowly comes through your ears and into your eyes. Your eyes have a filter that keeps you from seeing truth or reality because of the karmic lessons you need to complete here.

See the light from the stars of David coming into your eyes and washing away the filter. Visualize a small ray coming into your eyes. Hear the whispers of the rays washing through your eyes. You may feel some discomfort, perhaps some anxiety, as something is removed. Release it, and let it be washed away.

The energy comes out through your nose. Just allow this to happen. Let your ears send the energy into your eyes, wash your eyes, and then breathe it out through your nose. After everything has been released, transmute it into golden particles of light, and send it into Mother Earth's body.

By doing this exercise, you will learn to clearly see who you are. A shift will happen in your base chakra, and you will release the eight life-lesson patterns you brought here to master. Then you will be able to hear, see, and smell the truth of everything.

You can smell the truth. When you are near pets, a dog might smell you or a cat might rub up against you. What are these animals doing? They are sensing the truth of who you are. You will be able to do the same. Your nose will gain a heightened state of awareness, and you will be able to perceive energy by smelling it. It will have a very distinct smell.

Animals sense the truth of what they smell. You will develop this sense and use it in every situation and conversation. You will believe in yourself and your abilities, and you will transform your sense of unworthiness to high self-esteem as a being of light. I am Barbiel, the angel who supports feeling good about yourself. Good day and love to all of you.

✳   ✳   ✳

Archangel Michael here. We hope you enjoyed the conversation with Barbiel. We are ready for questions.

You had mentioned that Hanniel was the angel of happiness. Can you elaborate on the difference between Barbiel and Hanniel?

Hanniel also supports creating joy in your life, but Barbiel supports changing the energetic pattern inside you so that you start believing in yourself and then can feel joy. Hanniel supports the continual creation of joy, but joy must first be awakened. That happens through believing in yourself. Their roles are similar, but there is a distinct difference.

It starts with self-esteem?

Of course! Everything in life starts with self-esteem. You must feel good about yourself. Self-esteem is the basis of everything.

Is self-esteem the same as ego?

No. You must have an ego too. People put the ego down, but a controlled ego is important. Without ego, you cannot survive. The ego pushes you to excel in life, to reach beyond your limits. It is ego that says, "I can do better." Do not fight your ego. You cannot deny it; it is part of you. Work with your ego to create a higher reality for yourself.

Your false ego leads you to say, "I am better than others. I am special, and they are not." Use your ego for what it is meant, which is to help you rise to a higher reality. If the Wright brothers had not had egos, they might not have succeeded in making an airplane. All inventors have egos; it provides the motivation to create something better.

✳   ✳   ✳

Awaken Your Celestial Sense of Smell

Blessings, blessings, and blessings. We are El Varha, the angel of smell. Most human beings understand smell only through their noses. In reality, the nose is simply another tool. Smelling is done through the body with input from the brain.

Think again about pets and how they greet you. You say they are sensing when they sniff you or rub against you, which is true, but how do they sense? They sense through their bodies. Your body is your greatest tool. It has sensitive pores, and through them, your sense of smell is fully awakened. A cheetah or leopard can smell its prey from almost 4 kilometers [2.5 miles] away. They sit and twitch their noses, their bodies pick up the vibrational frequency of the animals they sense, and they discern that as smell.

You can develop what is called celestial smell, or smelling things that are beyond the human nose's ability to sense, in the same way. You might have heard stories of people who smell the scent of flowers and know Mother Mary is present. When you awaken your sense of celestial smell, you can smell other realities and make them parts of your everyday life. This will enrich your life.

Smells can help you remember. That is their purpose. When people smell freshly baked bread, most feel good because the scent triggers subconscious memories of happy times in childhood and brings those feelings into the present. It all happens in a nanosecond because the body understands the smell and remembers. When you are able to awaken your sense of celestial smell, your body remembers who you are, where you have come from, and where you are going.

Each plant has its own smell vibration. For example, sandalwood has the capacity to open the human mind and body to other realities. The smell of naturally grown moss has the potential to help you transcend your reality. Every plant has a different smell. Look at what smells support you. They can enrich your life.

Brother Mordechai lives in Jerusalem and goes to pray at the Wailing Wall. He places his head and nose against the wall. What is he truly doing? He is sensing the frequency embedded in the wall through his body. When you are conscious of this, your experience multiplies many times over. This is true not only of the Wailing Wall but also of many sacred places. When you are in a sacred place, you can sense and smell through your body, whether you are at the Great Pyramid or the red rocks in Sedona, Arizona, for example. You can consciously awaken your body's understanding of celestial smell.

Experience Celestial Smell through Your Body

Take an apple in each hand, and bring them to your nose to smell them. Then place the apples in a container and close it. Say, "I wish to experience the smell of these apples through my body." Initially, you may want to place your hand on top of the container. You will feel the essence of the apples coming into your body, and your sense of smell will be more awakened. At first, you might still use your nose, but you will also sense the vibration and smell through your body. You can do the same for water or other things.

Practice this exercise to open to your celestial bodies. Some say that your celestial bodies come from the origin of the galaxy. They are much more than that. They are all that is, all that was, and all that will ever be. You can develop your celestial bodies.

Each ascended master has a vibrational frequency and color and emits a celestial smell. When a master enters, you smell a scent, such as the essence of flowers for Mother Mary that was mentioned earlier. In your meditation, you can ask for these smells to be revealed. As soon as the master enters, you will smell the scent. This will not only affect your sense of smell but also your brain. There will be healing in your brain as a higher frequency of light comes into it.

You are all travelers on the journey of life. Everything has a frequency and vibration. Along with that, everything emits light and has a smell. Smell is a frequency, just as love is a frequency, and your body is very well adapted to understanding and accepting frequencies, for it is also a frequency.

Here is a mantra to say every day: "My body is vibrating at the celestial level. I am one with all celestial beings." Your understanding of your body will be at a very high level, and this mantra will increase its vibration.

Your liver can support the awakening of celestial smell. The liver is a very sensitive organ that is affected by many things, including your food and your thoughts. There are glands inside your liver that connect directly to the organ of smell. When your liver is fit, you become more sensitive to smell and can also block undesirable smells.

Try this exercise to strengthen your liver. It will help you block everyday worldly smells and slowly awaken celestial smells.

Breathe in from the left side of your body between your stomach and your heart, and exhale through the right side. Repeat this about ten times. Then breathe in from the right, and exhale from the left.

When you awaken to celestial smells, your intake of food shifts. Your body fills with higher vibrations, and you do not need to eat as much. You begin to feel well. You then awaken to higher love and all the higher qualities of the fifth dimension, such as compassion, kindness, love, and forgiveness. The universe emits a sound frequency and a smell at all times. Tune into it to feel its presence.

We encourage you to look at every aspect of your life as a vibration that you can cultivate, actualize, and use. The senses are there to support you. You might be using them only peripherally, but they can work more deeply through your body. We encourage you to examine smells that support you. Ask the masters and the angels of celestial smells to reveal those smells to you.

We encourage you to look at the fascinating world of smells. Look at why some things attract and others repel. Bees are attracted to flowers but not all flowers.

Enter the Rejuvenation Temples

In your meditation, you can ask to bring forth the heavenly smells of rejuvenation. It will be like manna for your cells. Call this forth, and it will be given.

How do cells rejuvenate, and how can you be strengthened? You could say through love or light, but you are more restored through smell. Of all the senses you have, smell works the fastest and is the strongest. It cuts through all the layers and goes deeply into your core essence. There are temples of rejuvenation on the inner planes. They strengthen your body, mind, and soul. Ask for the smell of rejuvenation. If you ask, it will be given to you.

Close your eyes and ask your soul to take you to the temple of rejuvenation. See yourself in this temple, and ask to be taken to the chamber of rejuvenation and the celestial bed of smells. Imagine lying on a bed with twelve fountains beneath it emitting twelve scents and bubbles of light in twelve colors into your body. These bubbles become silver and gold sparkles in sacred geometric patterns. This is a beautiful experience. Partake of this for several minutes. When you wake, thank the attendees who helped, and slowly open your eyes.

✳   ✳   ✳

This is Archangel Michael. Does anyone have a question?

It felt as if this was a portal to a book of secrets in our bodies.

Of course, and to the heart of God.

✳   ✳   ✳

How to Awaken Your Celestial Sense of Smell

This is El Varha. We would like to give you examples of how some scents can help you open your sense of celestial smell.

- Lily and lilac can help you release. Some people have difficulty releasing things — an object, a thought, a pattern, a behavior, a person, or an incident. Apply lily essence on the soles of your feet and behind your ears before you go to sleep. This can help you release gently without burdening your body. Some forms of release can bring forth sadness, anger, or bodily discomfort. When you release this way, you do not experience discomfort.
- Sage can help you clarify your thoughts. When you have clarified thought, you can have clarified communication. Green sage placed in the house can help clear thoughts. This can be purchased in the market, but try to buy it in its most natural form possible. A flower is best.
- The white-flowered jasmine has a very strong smell. It has been a temple flower in India, Sri Lanka, Thailand, and other countries

where they make jasmine offerings to the gods they worship. The smell of jasmine can invoke inner reflection, allowing you to look very deeply at your life and understand the divine within you.

- There are many different types of tulips. Pick one you like. The smell of tulip can help you release issues you might have with your mother or other women in your life.
- The smell of dandelion can help you understand and release issues you have with your father or other male figures.
- Calla lily is the flower of Master Hilarion. It can help you understand your connection with your guides and inner teachers. It helps you move forward in your spiritual growth.

We ask you to work with scents every day. You might say, "I awaken the celestial bodies within me," and connect with your celestial bodies throughout the space-time continuum. When you awaken your sense of smell, you also awaken other fine qualities, such as gentleness, grace, and joy. Are you ready to experience this magic? We, the angelic realm, will support you in this manifestation. Everything you know has a smell. When you connect with smell, you connect with something's core essence, its vibration. Good day to you. I am El Varha, the angel of smells.

❋　　❋　　❋

Heal and Rejuvenate through Breathing

Hello, my name is Sanhriel. I am the angel of air. In the dream state, every master breathes, but not always through the nose as human beings do. Everything in the universe breathes. The Creator breathes — in and out. It's important to understand breathing and how it can liberate you. Understanding the flow of air into the body is key. Most people are not aware of how the inflow of air affects them. They breathe automatically.

Breathing can be regulated to send oxygen to specific parts of the body. It can hold certain energies. Let us say you have malignant tissue in your body. By understanding the movement of air, you can stop sending it to a cancerous growth so that tissue does not have the nutrition necessary to continue growing.

You can also send energy through breathing to rejuvenate your tissue so that new growth can occur. After losing an arm, a starfish can produce a new one and become whole again. But human beings are not able to regrow parts of their bodies. How does this work? The key is understanding the air you inhale. If you work at breathing in and sending air to the parts of your body that need to grow and regenerate, you can, over time, achieve it.

Breathing techniques can help people with mental illnesses who are put in mental hospitals because society doesn't truly understand that the condition has a spiritual component. That condition is part of a person's blueprint, karmic work, and parents' karmic lessons. Such a person could be helped tremendously by breathing consciously and sending energy to the brain. A mental patient could truly help him- or herself by sending energy to the back of the neck. He or she would become more coherent and be able to understand what other people tell them.

Regulating air through the body is the key to many kinds of transformation and rejuvenation. People practiced body rejuvenation in ancient Atlantis and Lemuria. They used tools such as sound, colors, and symbols, but they also used breathing. Here we are taking breathing to the next level, sending your breath to parts of your body that need healing or rejuvenation.

A person who has cancer might have tried everything, but if he or she is willing to work, some improvements could be seen depending on his or her faith, self-confidence, and the technique used. There would definitely be improvement. I wish to say goodbye at this time.

※　※　※

This is Archangel Michael. I will take questions.

Could you clarify what was said about cancer and how breathing could be used to heal it?
People with illness must focus and send the energy that they breathe to the tissue containing the sickness. They must focus on both their breath and their awareness. They will see some differences if they do it regularly several times a day combined with the belief and faith that this is effective.

Open Your Vocal Cords

Welcome to the joyous celebration of life. When like-minded lightworkers join together and share light, love, and warmth, we enjoy this gathering.

When people gather, there is much brighter light. You can collectively send this bright light to any place in the world before or after the session. There is an energy buildup. This energy is pure and powerful, so you will be able to direct it to any part of the world. The first angel who would like to speak today is the angel Vohumanah. This angel is the angel of good voice.

*　　*　　*

Blessed one, we are the Angel Vohumanah. We have never spoken to a human being. This is our first experience speaking with an Earth being.

We support the vocal cords of human beings. Many people incarnate on the Earth plane with closed vocal cords because they have heavy karmic energy and life lessons that they have come here to master. They are often not able to speak clearly or lovingly or to express their truth or how they feel. When the vocal cords are blocked, the heart, the solar plexus (the point of power), and the second chakra are obstructed. Your vocal cords closed in past incarnations because you were ostracized, criticized, banished, or even killed when you spoke the truth.

The vocal cords are not only for speaking but also for bringing forth specific understandings and creative power. It is through the vocal cords that the soul expresses what it wants to manifest. You often see people who have problems speaking in the presence of authority. Their vocal cords close because of their fear. They are completely silenced.

You send commands to your brain through your vocal cords. You have a signature cell in your brain. It sends a command to all the cells in your physical body. When the vocal cords are shut, you are unable to communicate properly with the signature cell to send a command to carry out the manifestation process. You are not able to create what you want. The way you say something is very important because your body hears everything your voice says. When your vocal cords shut off, you are not able to express what you want in your life.

The process of creation involves opening the vocal cords so that you are very clear. When the vocal cords are clear, most people understand what they want to create and how they need to go about achieving it. However, many people are not aware of what they want to create even when they are in their sixties, seventies, and eighties.

What is the meaning of good voice? Good voice is the voice of God coming through you, the voice of tolerance, compassion, and love. When you start expressing these feelings — compassion, truth, and tolerance — through your voice, you use your vocal cords for their highest purpose.

Remember, in your world, most people are motivated by self-interest alone. It is rare for people to move beyond self-interest. However, they must begin to do things for the overall good of humanity. That can only happen when the vocal cords are open.

When your vocal cords are open, your eyes become very bright. You can see clearly, and the perceptive ability of your brain also opens. You see people as not only other human beings but also extensions of yourself. What you do to others, you do to yourself. Your voice has a very important role in helping you make this shift. This is why many traditions have breathing techniques to open the voice cords.

Many sounds can emerge from your vocal cords: The sounds of tolerance, compassion, and love are virtues of God. At the other end of the spectrum, hatred can also come forth through the vocal cords. When you speak through the voice of God, this affects every part of your body, from your eyes to your ears to your kidneys to the soles of your feet. All are energetically connected to your vocal cords.

Open the Good Earth Voice

Close your eyes, and bring your attention to your vocal cords. Make the intention to open the God voice within you. Visualize a beautiful clear white light in your throat. Let your throat be filled with that beautiful white light. See it go into the back of your neck and then flow into the back of your body to your hip area, the soles of your feet, and then the ground. Visualize a red lotus with four petals slowly open in your throat. A light emits from the center of this lotus. It goes into your face and your crown and then flows from your crown.

Now visualize a beautiful blue light coming from above into the middle of the lotus. This is a healing light from the Pleiadian brothers and sisters. Visualize this light shining through the petals and deep into the roots of the lotus, which are anchored at your third chakra. From there, the light flows through your kidneys. The kidneys are very important. They are part of your consciousness. When your kidneys are functioning properly, light will shine from them. This light is sent to your brain. See the blue light anchor into your solar plexus and from there, transfer to your kidneys, go into the back of the body, and anchor into the ground.

Ask that the good earth voice be opened unto you — good earth, good earth, good earth voice be opened unto you. Visualize a beautiful golden green light coming from the ground slowly enter your feet and move up into your solar plexus and then into the vocal cords. Visualize it soothing and bathing your vocal cords, filling them with golden green light. Let it flow, and give intent for it to also go into your auric field. See the golden green energy come into your auric field. Let this energy flow throughout your being. Let it all flow through you. You are bathed in this light.

When your vocal cords are closed, your aura will contain blocked energies. When your auric field is blocked, your consciousness is also blocked because your mind exists in your auric field. Your aura, along with your DNA, contains your history. When your vocal cords are clear, your ears will be clear. Your sense of perception will become very clear.

When you wake up in the morning for the next several days, state this intention: "I awaken the good earth voice within me. I anchor the energy of the good earth voice in my solar plexus and in my vocal cords." In a few days, this will become part of your reality. The way you speak will shift, and you will know when to speak, when to withdraw, and what to say. Your close friends will recognize that something shifted in you. You will be on the road to recovery. Blessings, I am Vohumanah, the angel of good voice, the voice of God.

✳ ✳ ✳

See Beauty to Find God

Hello, my family. This is Angel Yahoel. I am an aspect of Archangel Metatron. Under this name, Archangel Metatron teaches about righteous living, grace, and beauty. What does righteous living mean? All cultures talk about righteous living, which is living fully, gracefully, joyously, enthusiastically, and passionately.

Today I wish to talk about the beauty of life. There is great beauty in life, but many fail to observe it because they focus on a distant goal or the ancient past. They fail to recognize the beauty all around them. This beauty can support you during times of great stress or change.

Beauty can come in any form. Watch a child chasing a bird, a young boy flying a kite, a young girl jumping into a pool and shaking with happiness, a turtle taking a nap on a sunny afternoon, a flower blooming, or a dragonfly hovering in the summertime. There is beauty everywhere if you open your eyes to it. We encourage you to see, because the observation of beauty can bring balance and calm to your life. You are so focused on the outside that you forget to see the inner beauty or the beauty of a rainbow or a blue sky.

When you pass away after you finish your earthly life, these moments of beauty will be permanent impressions on your soul. You will look back fondly at the blue sky and say, "It was magnificent! There was so much beauty, and I missed it." These moments when you found, felt, and experienced beauty are etched in the memory of your soul. What you did, how you did it, or how much you did do not matter. The moments you recognize incredible beauty and feel the perfection of life will be etched into the memory of your soul.

We encourage you to look for beauty. Make it a point every day. Say, "Today I will seek beauty, and I will see beauty for at least five minutes." You could say, "I am a very busy person. When I get up in the morning, I have to get ready and go to work. I am rushed." Even in that, you can find beauty. Find it in a delicious cup of coffee. When you drive your car, appreciate the crisp early morning air or a soft breeze in the afternoon. Everywhere there is beauty.

Beauty is a quality of God. It has a very high frequency. Because you are a quantum being, a high frequency of light can penetrate to the deepest parts of your being and transform you. Can you imagine holding a vision of beauty within yourself for five minutes? What could that do for you? Your cells could understand it. They would start seeing beauty because you just commanded your cells with this high-frequency energy. Even on a dull, gray day during the coldest winter, learn to see beauty. Is a bird singing? What is your pet doing?

It is said that there are more than 3,000 beautiful experiences you can have in a given day if you choose to see them. However, you seldom focus on seeing beauty. We encourage you to do so. When you see beauty in your life, it is called righteous living. You will live in grace, appreciation, gratitude, and the truthfulness of who you are.

The energy of beauty is stored in your kidneys and sexual organs. When you are in love, you only see beauty in your lover, especially during the first few months. Both men and women can connect with the energy of beauty in your sexual areas. Ask for the energy of beauty to be awakened and expressed through your emotions.

Close your eyes, and bring your awareness to your sexual organs. Rest your attention there. Simply say, "I ask the energy of beauty to be awakened within me and that this energy flow through my entire being into the meridians, into my bloodstream, into my bones, into my skin, and into my hair." Just allow for this energy to flow through you.

When you work with the energy of beauty, you start to see only beauty in others, and you become a bridge. Beauty is God. God is beauty. Experience beauty through your emotional body. See God in everybody, and see the beauty within each person. Blessings, blessings, blessings. I am Yahoel, angel of righteous living, beauty, and grace.

CHAPTER TWO

Boost Your Mental Faculties

Angel Gidongh, Angel Sanyaso, Angel Kabriel, and Angel Val Na Thali

We are Angels Gidongh and Sanyaso. We are the angels of the internal and external minds, which are distinct and separate. Your internal mind processes what you have collected from other realities and the past, whereas your external mind processes information in your current reality. These two minds work together to bring you the perfect energy to work out your karmic and life lessons, or why you have come here.

Your internal mind has much more influence than your external mind because the internal mind is connected to your past. You must realize that there are many levels to your mind. You have heard about your unconscious mind, subconscious mind, supraconscious mind, and omni-mind. There is also the mohatmic mind. But for the purposes of karmic interactions and the lessons you have come here to master, you use only three levels of your mind: the subconscious, unconscious, and sometimes the supraconscious — but not all the time. You rarely venture into the other aspects of your mind. Your mind exists in all the other aspects too, but they lie dormant.

For example, perhaps you walked with Archangel Metatron in other lifetimes. This is stored in your higher mind. You will open this higher aspect of the mind, and when that happens, your outer mind will naturally become a part of this.

✳   ✳   ✳

Open to Codes of Higher Intelligence

Hello. I am Kabriel, the angel of higher intelligence. Have you ever wondered why some people have a higher IQ than others? Is it hereditary? What factors determine why some IQs are very high or why some people have higher intelligence than others? Some parents were poor and never went to school, but one of their children might be very bright. Where did that child get this intelligence? Is it a reflection of the child's karma? Yes, the first step is karma, but what happened in past lives? How can this person's consciousness have such high intelligence? Most important, can this open in you?

The answer is yes. Some cultures understood this. Ancient Rishis taught expectant mothers to take a small amount of ghee every day in the early morning to increase the possibility of having a child with high intelligence. There is a code inside your body (in your palms) for higher intelligence, and it can be activated.

Focus on where your wrist joins the palm. This is a very important place. It is the place used by the dark forces to control human beings. Etherically, they tie your hands there. When people are arrested, their wrists are tied. Subconsciously, this ties their intelligence so that the arrested people cannot think clearly, and somebody else thinks for them. When your higher intelligence is not awakened, you can be easily manipulated by the thoughts of others — a group, a teacher, or a dictator who speaks eloquently or boldly. Advanced students such as you who are on a path of ascension must awaken to your higher intelligence by focusing on this point.

Close your eyes, bring your awareness to your palms and wrists, and breathe from there. Breathe, and imagine holding a golden boat in your cupped hands. There are no oars, just a boat. Breathe, and see the boat rock back and forth, as if it were on ocean waves. As the boat rocks, you see explosions of light coming into it from the motion. The light enters the middle of your palms and goes to your fingers. Lightly press your fingers on both eyes, and send this energy through your eyebrows. It goes though your whole body and into the other realities you inhabit.

Keep doing this. As the golden boat rocks back and forth, energy comes into the boat and moves from the boat into your hands, into your fingers, up to your eyes, through your eyebrows, and into other realities. Allow this process.

The energy from your eyebrows slowly begins to flow into your brain, to the back of your head, to the ascension chakra at your medulla oblongata, and then through your spinal column and into your hips. Your hips are an important receptor for energy. Many karmic energies saturate and concentrate there. See the light go down into your hips, making them feel lighter. See them being filled with light and becoming loose and saggy. They have lost the condensed energy that kept them so tight.

Place your hand on your hips and say, "I release. I love. I know. I experience. I am." When you heal your hips, you will heal a lot of issues in your mind. You will be liberated. You will have freedom. "Freedom" is another word for God.

We encourage you to do the exercise for the next twenty-one to forty days, and you will see your intelligence open like a beautiful flower. A new way of thinking, understanding, and experiencing will open to you. You will be amazed by what you can bring forth. You can call on me: "Kabriel, support me in this."

What is higher intelligence? Simply stated, it is the ability to perceive a new truth. With higher intelligence, you can see a potential reality within your being. Higher intelligence, when followed with appropriate action, can change the world. When it is awakened, you break the shackles of those who control humanity. You will be able to stand in a new reality and a new truth.

We thank you for the opportunity to speak with you today. It is through Archangel Michael that we experience this interaction.

❈   ❈   ❈

Combine and Integrate Your Subconscious, Unconscious, Supraconscious, and Omni-Minds

Blessings, blessings, blessings and love to all. I am Val Na Thali. I have been given this undertaking to help human beings and other kingdoms (plants, animals, minerals, stones, oil, and so on). All have consciousnesses on different levels, just as you have different consciousnesses on different levels. They are also in their own evolutionary processes. For example, a stone must evolve further in its stone time. If not, it would disintegrate and once again become the elements from which it was created. Everything in the universe must evolve in its own time. A mountain is evolving all the time. A young mountain has peaks, and when it matures, it becomes like a mound. Everything evolves — everything.

I support the evolution of all that I mentioned. Each has different levels of consciousness. A plant has at least three layers of consciousness: plant consciousness, deva consciousness, and God consciousness. Plants have personalities and souls.

Human beings have many layers of mind, but the most important layers you must work with are the subconscious mind, the unconscious mind, the supraconscious mind, and the omni-mind. If not controlled and checked, your unconscious and subconscious minds will rule your life and often ruin it. What do I mean by ruin? Your unconscious and subconscious minds contain thought processes from past realities. These are often from not only you but also your ancestors, culture, and your heritage from long ago. Cleansing the subconscious mind is very important.

Many people talk about clearing the subconscious mind, but it is not that easy to do. If it were, everyone would have done it. There are certain processes that can support you in bringing your subconscious mind to a much more fertile place where you will be able to plant seeds so that healthy plants can grow.

The subconscious mind has a spectrum of colors, and each layer of consciousness has a different color. The color of the subconscious mind, where thoughts are nurtured and then pushed forward to manifest in physical reality, is a soft green. Your unconscious mind is directly connected to your subconscious mind but is more evolved. It has a soft metallic blue color. The supraconsciousness, or superconsciousness, layer has a color frequency of gold with sacred geometry inside it. The geometry is a golden wheel with twenty-four spokes. The omni-mind is a beautiful turquoise. It also has a sacred geometric pattern: two seeds cut in half and placed side by side.

Close your eyes and envision these four colors: soft green, soft metallic blue, gold with a twenty-four spoked wheel, and turquoise with two seeds cut in half. Breathe into these colors and see them slowly shift position. See the four colors slowly blend. The supraconscious mind starts spinning. You can see all the colors go into the golden wheel, and the wheel spins. Let it spin. The wheel becomes larger and larger. Let it become bigger than you. It is spinning at a very high frequency. Allow it to spin faster and faster. You slowly disappear. There is only the wheel. Allow this to continue.

See this wheel become smaller and enter your tenth chakra one arm's length above your head. As it spins, it flows through your pranic tube in the middle of your spinal column. There are strings on the back of your spinal column that go into the front of your body, and they start spinning, making a loop back to your pranic tube. The wheel flows down into your legs and spins there. Then it comes up again, making another loop. The two loops interconnect.

The spinning circle slowly stops. Breathe into this stopped circle. A new color slowly emerges from this. The color will be different for each person. Breathe into this new color. See the color flow into the colors you started with — green (the subconscious mind), metallic blue (the unconscious mind), and turquoise (omni-mind). Those colors are no more, and there is only your new color. Breathe into that.

Allow the new color to flow through your feet, and release it into the ground and into your toes. Toes are very important. The big toes hold the wisdom of Mother Earth in your physical body. This energy is going into the toes so that from now on, every step you take doesn't just come from your unconscious, subconscious, supraconscious, or omni-mind but a combination of all.

Raise the energy to your toes, and anchor it there. Breathe it in and simply say, "I give intention to hold this new frequency within me from today onward. I am joined in all my minds, all my consciousness, all my energy." Breathe in deeply.

The next time you want to activate this energy, bring your attention to your toes and your feet, and simply say, "I activate the new consciousness of my combined minds." Breathe it in three times, focusing on your feet, and you will feel the energy shooting out. Breathe once again and once again and once again. Slowly open your eyes.

❋　❋　❋

This is Archangel Michael. Your aura and manifestations have become very powerful. When you work with this meditation, be aware that your mind can become very powerful. Thoughts you hold have the potential to manifest immediately for the next several hours or days. Be very clear what is in your thoughts because this is God power within you, the power of your mighty I Am presence.

CHAPTER THREE

Expand Your Consciousness

Archangel Michael, Angel Tenariel, Angel Eth, Archangelic Essences,
Angel Oriel, and Angel Yahadriel

This is Archangel Michael. As you raise your vibration, you raise the vibration of the planet and the place where you live. No matter what challenges happen in the world, your homes will be protected. I offer this humble gift to my brothers and sisters of the light. Ask me to place the sword of truth in one of your hands and the sheath of wisdom in the other, for these will be your new walking sticks. These will make you courageous and allow you to believe in yourself — in your ability to stand on your own and, most importantly, to know that you are a master.

At some level, most humans know this, but they do not believe it. Since they do not believe it, they are not able to walk that truth. My shield and sword will remove the energetic codes that prevent you from believing, experiencing, and being the master you truly are.

In your meditations, you can also ask me to activate the Michael code within you. When you activate the Michael code, you activate my essence within your being, and I become a part of you, always inside you. The energies of all the masters are inside every human being, but they are dormant unless you activate the codes. Think of your home with rooms wired for electricity. Electricity runs through the wires, but the rooms remain dark unless you flip the switches. It is similar with our energy. The consciousnesses of all the masters and angels who are a part of your support group exist within you, but you must call them forth and activate the codes. This is my gift to all of you at this time. Blessings.

Activate Love

Dear Earth brothers and sisters, we are the energy of the angel of love. We are a group energy, and our name is Tenariel. We can support you in many ways to fully understand and practice true love. We can help you mend a broken heart or find a life partner, for it is the desire of the Creator that human beings grow through partnership because it offers much learning and growth. If you sincerely seek a partner with whom you can couple and enjoy the totality of another human being and through that person discover more of yourself and of God, you can call on us. We impart energy, wisdom, and understanding about the true nature of love.

Love can never be fully explained. It can only be experienced. This experience depends on each person's evolution and where he or she is in life.

True love is silence. It is felt, on an energetic level, coursing through your cellular structures. People say, "I am in love" when they have certain feelings, but thoughts often masquerade as feelings. True love is silence.

There are also many nuances of love, such as when to share it, when to express it, and sometimes when to withhold it — not because you do not want to share, but because you want to bring an understanding to the person who might need to experience that withholding.

There are many aspects of love. One important aspect is that it cannot be contained. Love is All That Is. If God is All That Is, God cannot be contained in any way. It is the same with love. It can never be contained. You can choose to spend long periods with one person if you choose to experience love from one source, as in a marriage or a relationship. However, this is only part of the truth, for true love can never be contained.

Perhaps you were in love at certain times in your life. Although you went through this experience and forgot about it, that flame remains a part of your energetic field. You can reconnect with that soul any time through the energetic pattern you already hold, especially if that love was based on purity, sacredness, and divinity.

Does love mean you have to share everything? This is an individual choice. You do not have to. Once love is open, it can never be extinguished. You can choose to say, "I can completely put it down," but like a box containing a coiled spring, as soon as you open it, love expands.

There is also love between a mother and a child, between family members, or between a person and a flower, an animal, or a beautiful landscape. When you work with us, we bring an understanding of how all the different aspects of love can be combined so that you see only love in every human being you encounter. When that happens, you see God in every human being. This is the ultimate aim of human life. People might have imperfections, but the spark of God exists in their hearts, and you can see and feel that spark. You realize they might have forgotten who they are because they are exhibiting a part of themselves that is not of God or love, but when you can see God in everyone, you have great compassion. This is the love of God.

Close your eyes, bring both your palms to your heart, and gently breathe from your heart. When you breathe out, visualize a beautiful soft purple color slowly coming out of your hands. Breathe normally, and when you exhale, the soft purple comes out of your fingers. Soft purple is the color of true love. It is a vibrational color. True love is a vibrational frequency that you experience on the cellular level, and when you exhale this color, you will be able to experience love coming out through your hands and going out to the world. Anytime you feel you need an extra dose of love or you forget that you are love itself, do this simple exercise for three to five minutes. You will awaken to the inner knowingness that you are a being of love.

The Code of Love

What happens when you die? After a certain process of energy assimilation, you rejoin the incredible force of love. You may call it by any name: spirit, unified intelligence, energy, or whatever. It is not white. It is soft purple. You are immersed in that color. Master Saint Germain works with the flame of transformation, and it is the same color. When a human being is born, the birthing angels place a soft purple dot in the solar plexus of the baby, and this energy slowly transmits its frequency to all cells. The child is very pure and has not forgotten who it is when it is born. The frequency emitted from this dot is very pure, and everyone feels love from the child. However, after time and conditioning, this energy closes off. You can ask that the code of love that was placed by the angels during your birth be fully activated inside you.

Place your hands on your solar plexus, and visualize a sphere emitting a beautiful soft purple light. Breathe it in, and immediately feel a surge of love within you. This sphere is directly corded to the chakras underneath the soles of your feet. When you activate this energy, it goes into the ground and helps other people and Mother Earth. What a beautiful creation, how the Creator put this together! It is now time to awaken this energy and the code of love within you in your solar plexus.

When you work with this energy daily, you will understand love mentally and experience all the nuances of love in your physical body. You will open yourself to new realities from the other side through which beings of light can communicate with you, including those from the tenth, eleventh, and twelfth dimensions. They see that you activated the code of love, and they can see you as the shining star you have become.

How do masters see a human being? They see you as a twinkling star. They see the emanation from the star and the frequency of light you hold. It is very safe for us to communicate at that level. This soft purple is called the velvet code within the solar plexus. Masters and angels know it right away. They know that you are in the beginning stages of fully integrating the God force within you, truly stepping onto the path of ascension and being a master of love.

You may call me when you want to couple with another human being who shares the same values as you and through whom you can share life and increase your joy. I offer this in humble gratitude. I am Tenariel, the velvet angel of love.

❋ ❋ ❋

This is Archangel Michael. When we have a benevolent and loving partner, life is so much richer. A true partnership is a treasure more valuable than all the money you could ever have. It can bring beauty and incredible joy. When you have love in your life, you experience a great shift.

People who hurt others do not have love in their lives for another human being, an animal, or nature. When there is no love, people shut off their emotional bodies and are not able to feel anything. They shut out not only love but all other emotions as well. They are not able to feel much of anything. They become like robots.

When people join the military, part of the emotional body shuts down. These people join the military because it is in the life blueprints they formed in other lifetimes to break the predisposition for becoming a soldier. They often come together in the same unit. Their life missions are to break the chain of violence.

Activate Time Codes

We are honored to speak with the angel of time, Eth. This angel is another aspect of Archangel Metatron. Metatron wears many hats.

You have heard a great deal about time. There is no linear time. There is circular time, not "this" time or "that" time. If you want to get a grip on time, we encourage you to look at time differently.

❋   ❋   ❋

Blessed family, it's a privilege to speak with you at this gathering of beautiful souls. We are the energy of Eth.

Your understanding of time can shift. You can look at time as vertical, or moving up and down. We can call "moving up" the future and "moving down" the past. Do you move time? If you were to look at your life and say, "I want to move through the vertical aspects of time," then you would remember your future and your past. Your future already exists in one reality. You say that it has not happened yet, but since you have simultaneous realities at once, your future is created at this time. It exists.

There is a time code in your physical body. It is behind your neck. You can ask to activate this time code to help you accomplish various things. You could set the time code for your ascension in three years. It would be like an alarm clock, and at that time, it would start ringing within you. You could set the time code to complete a book or get married by a certain time. You can work with time, and it will support you energetically to create what you want to create.

Often your reality is not created in accord with what you want to create. You may have tried many times. If time does not support something, it will not happen. This is why it is said that everything has divine timing. When you activate the time code in the back of your neck, everything happens with divine timing in the present moment of reality. Your mind will only create that which is the highest good for you in that moment. Time becomes your friend.

You can set your time code by saying, "Today I give intention to stop the process of aging in my cells. This aging process was an old, past timeline. I disconnect from this past timeline." You could say, "I set my timeline in the next three years to look younger and to have energy of a younger person but with the wisdom of my present years." Time will work with you. You will have more energy and a younger appearance, but your wisdom will still be with you.

The Universal Time Code

You can also ask that the universal time code inside your crown chakra be fully activated. You can call on the Andromedan masters to recalibrate and reset this universal time code within your head.

Gently close your eyes, and bring your attention to the top of your head. Call on the great masters of Andromeda. Visualize a powerful beam of white light slowly coming into the center your head.

Ask the Andromedan masters to reset and recalibrate the universal time code in your brain. They are similar to body technicians and will do some rewiring. Once this is done, envision a golden beam of light coming from the center of the universe and flowing into your brain. This is a beautiful tube of golden light. You may feel sensations in your eyes, your third eye, and your face as this energy slowly descends into your physical body.

When you activate the universal time code, you adjust your consciousness to the twelve different times in which you exist in the universal reality. The other planets where you live have different times compared to the time frequencies of Earth. They do not look at time like you do. So you will recalibrate with the other twelve times in the other realities.

Your understanding and your energy will shift. There will be greater awakening within you. Some of you might have feelings of levitation. You might feel as if magnetics and gravity have diminished. You might feel as if you can move slowly above the ground. This is just one aspect of time. Blessings, I am Eth, the angel of time.

❇   ❇   ❇

Integrate Archangelic Energies

We are the essences of Archangels Metatron, Michael, Raphael, and Gabriel. We encourage you to call on our archangelic presence and integrate these energies into you. Just allow it. You might not see anything, but you will be able to sense it. Try to feel Metatron and Michael above you, Gabriel on your right side, and Raphael on your left side. Allow our energy to flow through you. The frequency of your energy will increase, for the greatest power lies with the archangels.

Most miracles are created by angels and archangels. Bringing these archangels into your life can boost your energy level. Our vibrations are very high, so you might also want to call on the spirits of the elements to ground their energies.

Because our energy can be quite strong, eat healthily. We encourage you to do this for several days until our energy becomes part of you. You can do your own ceremony to invite us into your home so that we become part of your environment there. We are the essences of the archangels.

✳   ✳   ✳

Open High Frequency Knowledge within You

I am Angel Oriel. Your body contains the Book of Secrets. In ancient Scotland, they called the body the Book of Secrets. Through the body, you can access higher vibrational frequencies and wisdom from the ancient past. I am speaking of a cell that developed long before this lifetime. The origin of this cell is ancient, and it might have germinated in another reality.

There is a perpetuation of cells during each birth. This happens when children of light are born. They carry the pure essence of the vibrations from their original frequencies, and they are able to bring it back. In many ways, cells are like clones. They carry their original vibrational intention and frequency, but these are often overshadowed by belief systems and thoughts. At the deepest level, these cells contain the original blueprint and code of God. When you get in touch with your body through your fingers, your toes, your eyes, and elsewhere, your body remembers that there is a true code, the original Book of Life.

Focus your attention on your upper back beneath your neck, and simply ask that the Book of Secrets be revealed within you. You might perceive a door opening and light pouring from it, inviting you inside. When you see the doorway, go through it to the deepest part of you. You will be led into the Hall of Records, which are in every human being. There you will see yourself as an ancient, wise spirit.

We also encourage you to open the Book of Records within you.

You are the universe itself. You have been told before that the universe exists within you. This is the meaning, for you are everything, and the Book of Records contains everything. Many have mentioned the Book of Records. We hope to awaken your thirst to find it. Many have searched unsuccessfully. It is inside you at the back of your body.

Start the process of connecting with your Book of Records through your fingers. The entire blueprint of your life is condensed in your fingers. To access your Book of Records, close your eyes and touch the tips of the four fingers of your left hand to the palm of your right hand. You will feel energy vibrations as you do this. Now slowly make clockwise circles with the fingers of your left hand in your right palm. Focus on your third eye. Your inner vision will open, and you will have clarity. You will have courage in your life. You will know what to do and how to proceed with the decisions you have to make. You will have answers at that moment not only about what decision you have to make but also about the consequences of all your decisions. It is all there. You will know how much energy to spend making a decision, whether you need to spend more energy on it or pull back, or whether you need to do a certain amount of work to create a specific reality. All will be revealed to you.

This is a secret code. It is only given when a student is ready. You are all ready to access this. By accessing this record, my teacher Elijah realized who he was, that he was God. On his appointed time, he went to the field for his own journey into the wildness.

Get in touch with your Book of Records, for it was written by you, the Creator. My love and blessings to all of you. I am the Angel Oriel.

❋   ❋   ❋

Experience the Creator through the Rising Sun

Blessings, brothers and sisters. I am Yahadriel, the angel of morning. Thank you for the opportunity to communicate with you. We thank Archangel Michael for encouraging us to speak.

Morning is a very special time in angelic lore. We call it the glory of God. The rising of the Sun is a celebration of God. It is a time of magic and miracles. If you can connect within yourself in the early morning, then you can see higher realities happen within you. This is especially true when you connect with the first rays of God, which appear at sunup. When you look at this sunlight, you can take energy from the experience. You can breathe it. You feel the energy coming into your nose, going through your mouth and deep into your intestines, and settling in your base chakra. Your base chakra will start spinning, and you will be filled with light. Then your experience will be from a higher reality, not from a wanting reality of "I need to survive, so I need. I want."

Close your eyes. Visualize the rising Sun, a beautiful white-orange, and see the rays coming into your nose and mouth and then filling your base chakra. Your base chakra starts to spin with this beautiful white-orange color, and this flows through your hands and legs into the ground. Just breathe it in.

This glorifies the Creator. What does glorifying the Creator mean? When you live your life fully from the base chakra, you live God, for life is God and God is life. You are not in a place of fear or want. You are in a place of celebration, and you have the opportunity to experience the Creator in everything you do and create that day. This is spirituality in a waking state.

You do not have to do anything to experience this. You will experience the highs and the lows, the joy and the sadness, and everything that life has to offer in its fullness coming from the place of fullness within you. You are simply living as God, fully present in every experience.

People sometimes think God cannot be sad and can only be positive. We say everything is God, for there is nothing that is not God. Experience every aspect of every day from the perspective of fullness. Come to this place every day. When you start your day with this practice, you are liberated because you are fully immersed in life.

Look at the masters. Masters never give everything up. They experience life fully in all that it has to offer. They reject nothing. They embrace it, and they call this liberation.

Call on me, the angel of morning, to support you in this. I work with twelve beings of light. There are twelve points in the physical body. You anchor light starting at the back of the head and then moving to the shoulders, the hips, the wrists, the toes, the knees, the earth beneath your feet, your auric field, your mental body, your emotional body, and your spiritual body. You will then start to live a celestial life. Your day will go well because you started it with light. You can experience everything each day through this light. You will not take things too seriously, for you know there is nothing to be too serious about. Even if something looks dense and heavy, it can melt in the light that you carry, and life will become play. This is why masters laugh a lot, for life is play. Unconsciously, you are playing. Blessings. This is the angel of morning, Yahadriel.

CHAPTER FOUR

Use Numbers to Improve Your Life

Archangel Michael and Angel Samariel

This is Archangel Michael. Numbers have a very important role in life. The magnetic master, Archangel Kryon, talks about numerology. The Maya understood the importance of numerology. Lemurians and Atlanteans understood the purpose of numerology and numbers. There is an angel, Samariel, who is the master of numbers, and we wish to bring him forth today. Most of the angels coming through have never spoken to human beings, but they are aware of Earth's important role. This is the first time this angel will speak to you.

✳ ✳ ✳

My dear brothers and sisters of this beautiful Blue Jewel, my name is Samariel. I hold the patterns and the movements of the stars for human beings, plants, and animals.

After a baby is born, it takes months before it can roll over and lie on its stomach and even longer to sit up, stand, and start walking. Similarly, a seed might take days or even weeks to grow after it is planted. Everything is in rhythmic order. There is divine timing and a divine plan for everything, and this relates to numbers. You can understand the workings of the universe when you understand numbers.

There are rings of light inside your spinal column that are shaped like the coils of a spring. When the fluids in your spinal column move upward, this energy coil can be fully activated, and you can once again come into balance.

The Significance of the Numbers 0 to 9

The numbers 0 to 9 have a great significance in the human body. When you are conceived, you are a sphere, a beautiful circle — the eternal being. The number 1 is the totality of everything, and a singularity is born. This could also be interpreted as an aspect of God, or the One. Then the cell divides into two. It contains the energy of the Father/Mother God, or the vesica piscis. Three represents the connection to the holy trinity. Four represents the forces of the four elements in the body. Five represents the five senses through which you experience life. Six represents divinity, the God force. Seven represents understanding the sacredness and holiness of life. Eight represents understanding, completion, and new beginnings, or death and rebirth. You are dying and being reborn every moment. Finally, the number 9 represents the ability to understand spiritual principals and live your life through them.

Where are the geometric patterns of these numbers in your physical body?

- The sphere (0) is on the top of your head.
- Number 1 resides in the middle of the solar plexus.
- Number 2 is behind your heart and connects to the front of your heart.
- Number 3 is in your spinal column, the perfect trinity of balance.
- Number 4 is between the heart and the throat chakra.
- Number 5 is between the second and the third chakras.
- Number 6, the divine and sacred, is in the third eye but also in your first chakra.
- Number 7 is behind the shoulders on the back of the body.
- Number 8 is in the forehead.
- Number 9 is underneath the soles of your feet.

Your body is mathematical. The energies of numerology are contained within your being. In your meditation, you can strengthen the energy of any number. With the power of intention, you can bring light from your solar plexus, your heart, or your third eye into these numbers and see them come to life. See them vibrate, pulse, and spin at a high speed. This activates the energy of a number in that part of your body. This energy does not stay only there; it crisscrosses throughout your body, but the base remains in the place where you established it. Every part of your body is uplifted by the energy that comes from that place, following the principles of hologram technology: One part affects the whole. We encourage you to work with these numbers. We guarantee that you will quickly see a shift happen.

Use Numbers to Change Your Frequency

Suppose you want to break a bad habit. You can use the quality of the 3, which is complete harmony with body, mind, and soul, but here we are speaking of the entirety of your mind and soul, your I Am presence. You will be able to sustain the changes you want to effect. The Maya were very proficient in this. They worked with the numbers to bring healing to their physical bodies.

Visualize the habit that you want to change as a small dot. See this dot spinning in perfect harmony and dissolving. In about seven days, you will feel a slight shift inside of you. The energy of the habit will leave your physical, mental, and emotional bodies.

You can ask for a new, higher-frequency template to form inside you. This could be peace, self-confidence, or love for yourself, depending on the habit you want to break. See this new template, and see the number 3 streaming and being distributed throughout your body.

Again, you will see a shift in about seven days. You will feel uplifted because your body will have received the message and the new template. We encourage you to experiment with this. You can change your life.

Master numbers have special frequencies and are tied to the base numbers 1 to 9. Here are some master numbers: 11, 22, 33, 44, 55, 66, 77, 88, 99, and 111. You can call for the frequency of these higher numbers. For example, you could say, "I call for the frequency of the master number 22 to be fully anchored into my number 3 area [spinal column], and I fully blend this energy within my being." You will slowly feel a shift happen. A thought pattern could appear. Each person experiences this differently. You might be inspired to call for another number. We encourage you to work with this.

Moses worked with numbers when he went to the mountain and saw the burning bush. He was given the commandments, but why were there ten? It was not God who commanded. God does not command anybody. We see this as a commitment, an energy configuration that can support humanity.

Every country has a numerical code with which it connects to its sisters in other realities. You have a fifth-dimensional body in a higher realm. Every country has higher realities in other dimensions. They communicate and connect using the frequency of numbers that are transmitted from mountain ranges, which act as antennas to convey messages to other realities.

You can also heal Mother Earth's body by inscribing numbers into her heart. You could incorporate the number 666. Six is a very holy number, for it is the number of liberation. Mother Earth will be affected by the energy of this number.

Attune to the Master Number of Archangel Metatron

Each master has a number with a unique vibrational frequency. We encourage you to look for the numbers of the masters, and you will be uplifted. There are numbers to connect with Master Melchizedek. There is a number to connect with Master Jesus. You can easily connect with Master Jesus with love, and you can use these numbers to connect to higher realities. Archangel Metatron has a very special vibrational frequency number through which we can connect.

Close your eyes, breathe, and bring your attention to your heart area. I will repeat some numbers. See these numbers come into your heart and form a beautiful, shiny platinum circle of light. Keep your focus on your heart as you breathe deeply: 1, 0, 2, 8, 1, 7. See these numbers embedded in your heart area with spheres of light: 1, 0, 2, 8, 1, 7. Breathe these in, and see shiny platinum silver spheres of light fill you your entire being. These are the master numbers of Archangel Metatron.

You can connect with everything in the universe through numbers. However, before you connect with the numbers of other beings or the numbers of masters, work with the numbers in your physical body to heal old patterns and behaviors and to incorporate new ones that you want in your everyday life. When you are confident and feel the energy, start working with the numbers of masters.

CHAPTER FIVE

Principles for Examining Doctrine to Make Sound Decisions

Angel Raziel, Archangel Michael, and Angel Oriel

Hello, family. My name is Raziel. You may have heard about me in your Kabbalah. The great Rabbi Akiva spoke about me. He was a great being who had a direct vision of God.

When there is a correct understanding of doctrine, there will be no conflict. All conflicts arise because of different interpretations of doctrine. Each has various interpretations. Understanding doctrine is critical at this time. You live in a world of information overload. So much is available. How can you know whether a doctrine is correct? Here are two principles for evaluating them:

- Does the doctrine you are reading or studying bring you to your truth and your own direct connection to God?
- Does this doctrine contain the frequency of love in written form?

Earth's Level of Destiny

I am Archangel Michael. Sometimes you come to a crossroad in your life. You do not know which way to go, where to turn, what actions to take, or what choices to make. It can often be scary to simply envision what is happening because you are afraid of making a wrong decision that could lead to pain and suffering. In these situations, some people might not make a decision at all. Angel Oriel, the angel of destiny and predisposition, can help you establish the boundaries and show you the appropriate steps to take during moments of indecision. As you develop your spiritual light quotient, the inner voice you hear will become less subtle. You have to make decisions every moment of your life as to who you will be and what you will experience. Calling on this angel can support you in understanding the role and direction you must take.

* * *

My dear family of Earth people, I am the Angel Oriel. A human being has a destiny, a goal, and a set design. In a larger sense, the planet has a destiny and a goal that it is slowly moving toward. Like human destiny, the planet's destiny can shift and change depending on the consciousness of its people and the choices they make.

This planet has had many opportunities to reach its destiny, but it did not. It collapsed. Right now, Earth is in its fifth level of destiny, and this time there is a very high probability that it will reach its destiny. "Destiny" simply means a desired goal was set for the people and the planet before you arrived. A desired goal can be achieved by following a certain path or by taking a shortcut. You will eventually reach your goal, but it might take a hundred lifetimes, or it could take three. That is a choice, and this is where predisposition comes in.

At this time, because of the intense energies on the planet, human beings are forced to make changes, and sometimes those are through a strong hand beyond human means and control. Although many of you are aware that you have moved to a new consciousness, there is a lingering anxiety in people's hearts. You hear rumors about a financial meltdown. There is a sense of anxiety among people. What is happening? Everything seems out of control, and people feel helpless. Will the money system collapse in the United States? What is happening in China? Trillions of dollars have been lost. Will this affect other countries? Will what has happened in Greece have a domino effect on other countries?

In this time of uncertainty, you must decide what steps to take. You make choices every moment — what to eat, what to wear, when to bathe, when to brush your teeth. You make decisions every moment. How can all these little decisions take you to the larger goals you have set for yourself? The key question is this: Are your everyday decisions leading you to your life goals? We encourage conscious living, because without it, what you choose every moment does not take you to the goals you have set.

When you are confused or anxious, you might not know the best way to proceed.

Bring your attention to the areas between the middle of your palms and where your fingers join your hand. Breathe in through the soles of your feet, and exhale through the part of your hand where the fingers join the inside of the palm. Just breathe. You may feel a tingling sensation in that part of your body. Just keep breathing.

Suppose you want to make a decision. "Should I eat in this restaurant today?" "Should I take this trip?" "Should I go out with this person?" You are not sure whether the action is for your highest good or would bring you a desired result. Would it be part of the overall desired goal you want to achieve? Do the breathing exercise above. If your fingers tingle and you feel an expansion of energy, a feeling of warmth, or a sense of peace, then the activity is a positive thing for you to do. If you do not feel anything at all or have a feeling of emptiness, fear, or uncertainty, then perhaps you should decide not to proceed at this time. It may not be in accord with divine time. Everything has divine timing, and you can feel this through your base chakra and your solar plexus.

Let's say you face a decision. If now is not the appropriate time, and it would not bring you the appropriate lesson for you to master, or is not for your highest good — no matter how hard you try — it is very possible that you won't feel anything. Sensation will be delayed by the energies coming from the base chakra through the solar plexus. When you do this exercise, what you have come here to do must align with the divine clock inside you. This simple exercise, practiced every day, will help you make choices when you do not know what to do. Breathe in, and release your breath where your fingers and palms join inside the palm.

Every part of your body has a vibrational frequency and a special essence and quality. This is why it has been said many times to honor your body, for it is a temple.

CHAPTER SIX

Find Your Blueprint and Life Plan

Angel Zachariel, Angel Charhar, Angel Khalmauel, Archangel Michael, Angel Hritorhm,
Angel Nehur-Ra-Sim, Angel Sadha, Elija, Angel Scargohsa, and Angel Citrayomhei

Hello, dear family. I am the angel of creation. My name is Zachariel. Many angels work to support the creation process. We walk hand in hand with the Elohim who create forms, taking inspiration from the heart of the Creator. We are here to support the creation of a New Earth by creating a new reality in each person's life. If everyone could connect with all that he or she was born to create on the soul level, there would be no time for diversions or drama. Most people have forgotten their true purpose — why they were born and what they are here to create. They end up doing other things in their efforts to find purpose.

Creation has many forms. Where does creation come from? Where is it going, and who is going to benefit from it? You must look at all those aspects when you try to harmoniously create what you have come here to create. You may call on us for help. We can help you find, refine, or redefine your creative efforts.

Some people do many things but nothing of substance. They think they have had varied experiences and their lives grew richer because they have done so many things, but were they truly doing what they came here to do as part of their soul's blueprint and contract? When you call on us, we can help you define what you are doing and determine whether it is part of your contract. Then we can help you make your creation. It can be manifested more easily instead of through struggling.

There are three parts to creating the reality that originates from your soul: You use your mind, your emotions, and your passion. The passion code of creativity is in the back of your body, in the spinal column. Some people become more creative when their kundalinis awaken. They slowly enter into passion. You can ask that your passion code be activated. You will then use all your senses and your whole body to create what you have come here to create.

If you seek only abundance, will you also find peace or joy? Usually not. You often become afraid. Will your abundance last for years or into your next life? When you approach life from your passion, you no longer work. Your efforts become joyful creation. We can help you fine-tune your creative abilities and define the purpose you were born for.

Your everyday life provides many clues about your purpose and why you were born, but most people fail to see them. They look outside themselves. Make it your intention to look for the purpose of your life and to create what you have come here to do. Look for the clues in your life. If you were to observe your life and the time when you were born, you would see at least twenty clues to guide you to your chosen destiny.

We ask you to call on the angelic creation group energy of which I am a part. We work not only from the Earth level but up to the seventh and eighth dimensions. There are frequencies of light that we can download into human beings, into their backs and the backs of their hands. Most people use their hands and their voices to create. There are very specific energies in the back of the hands.

In DNA activation, one layer is called "unshackling the chains tied around your wrist" [or "opening the blind eye and seeing without illusion"]. When you are caught in illusion, you are unable to deliver on what you came here for, and you live a life of minimal existence because your power has been taken away. Focus on this. Call on the angels of creation, and we will download energies into you. You can also ask these angels to remove the "shackles" from your wrists so that you can return to your passion.

Enhance Your Creative Ability

Many people create because of fear. They think that if they do not create, they could end up having nothing and even become homeless, waiting for someone else to support them. Others create out of competition. They look at life as a game of chess and think they must win no matter the cost.

Most of you have experienced this. Some people create from their egos. "I can create. I am great because I have the capacity to create."

We will help you redefine what true creation is, and this can benefit you at the soul level as well as all of humanity. We will support you when you create and help you understand how your creation can benefit others. For example, some people have brilliant ideas but are not able to create in such a way that other people are aware of those efforts. We will help you attract the people who are part of your growth process to your creation.

You can use the energy of water to create a new reality. Write down three, four, or five things you intend to create. Fill a glass of water. Meditate in front of it, and say, "These are the things I wish to create in my life." After you meditate with the utmost feeling of love from your heart, sprinkle the water around the rooms and on the plants in your house. Drink the remaining water from the glass, and ask that your intentions go into your entire body. Your house will then carry the energy of your intentions for your creative process.

Do this a few times. Your house has a spirit. Everything in your house is alive at the quantum level. The energies in your house will help you dream about what you need to do and how to create what you want.

You can also create using flowers. If you have flowers in your garden, go outside and communicate with the flowers after you meditate. Say, "I place with you the energy of my intention to create so that I can benefit along with others who are touched by my creation, and I offer this as a gift from my soul."

Invite the birds, the butterflies, and the bees. When they drink the nectar from the flowers, they will carry your intention and spread it to other flowers. Someone else can pick up the inspiration through what you created.

Simple things can help you create. We encourage you to consider this and ask for our support to manifest a desired reality, a creation coming from your soul. This is part of your soul blueprint. It will benefit you and others.

I am Zachariel. In your meditation, ask me to activate the passion code within you and remove the shackles from your hands and your vocal cords so that true power can once again return to these important places in your body. Blessings and great love to all of you.

* * *

Master the Eight Aspects of God

My name is Charhar. I am the angel of planning. You might wonder why I have come to speak with you today. Archangel Michael requested my presence. I am honored to be part of this group, an exalted group of light-workers. My specialty is to help you plan your life so that you can fully step into the reality of why you were born.

The Amish community knows about life planning. They have a simple formula — 5 + 4 + 3: Five months of the year are spent working to support themselves and to make money, four months on service to humanity, and three months on travel. They follow this tradition, and some hold a very high vibrational frequency because of such planning.

You can plan your life to maximize your spiritual advancement, growth, and understanding of why you are here. This can be very beneficial. The purpose of being born in the world is to find balance in every area. All the sections of life must balance. Think about how you spend each day. Where do you focus? There are eight aspects of your life you should focus on and balance:

- spirituality
- family
- health and well-being
- work
- abundance
- creation
- contribution to the world
- grace

A principle in feng shui is to have balance in these eight aspects. In true feng shui, a house is divided into eight corners. Strengthening the energy in each corner can bring benefit and balance. Look at whether you balance these eight aspects of your life.

Some people spend considerable time focusing on the light. This is good, but do not exclude the other aspects because they are also part of God. You have come here to master all aspects. Work with me to enhance each aspect and understand how you can balance them all.

Draw a circle. Divide it with eight spokes, and label each section with one aspect. Use a pendulum or dousing rod, and ask where you lack energy among the eight aspects. You will be shown where you need to put your effort because these aspects contain some of the life lessons you have come here to master.

The energy of these eight aspects is inside you in the middle of your belly button. Your belly button is a very important part of your body. Here you were once corded to your mother, the creator of your life.

Focus your awareness there, and see eight streams of light originate from it and encircle your body. Let them flow, going to your auric body and shooting energies from your navel to the universe. Breathe into this, and visualize a beautiful pyramid in the middle of your belly button. On top of the pyramid is a compass, and the compass is spinning. The compass stops at the section you must focus on.

"Focus" means give energy. There is an imbalance of energy in the aspect of your life where the compass pointed. Some people need to take personal time to nurture themselves. Others need to take action to manifest abundance. Some may write a book as part of their life contracts for their contribution to the world. You can ask the compass to turn again and to show you where you need to focus and balance your energy. The compass will move again. There is a compass inside your brain that correlates to the compass in your belly button, and a third compass exists beneath the soles of your feet. When the three compasses work in unison, you become a balanced being who is here to master your life.

In ancient times, ascension was different from today. Now ascension tests the balance of energy of these eight areas of everyday life. Eight is the number of completion. Before you go to sleep, ask that we work with you to help you further understand these aspects of your life. Then you can write a plan for what you need to do to achieve balance among them. When you focus on your belly button and work with the compass daily, you will make great strides. My name is Charhar, the angel of planning.

* * *

Attune to Your Divine Blueprint and I Am Presence

Dear family, we are the angelic presence known by the name Khalmauel. We are the angel of the body and coordination. As you know, every part of the body must coordinate with every other part to bring about the specific vibration and frequency for the whole body to function harmoniously. Ask yourself whether your body truly functions as it is supposed to and whether all parts work in coordination. You might say no because as your body's clock shifts and changes, its perfect pattern shifts as well. This affects the energy of the chakra column and the emotions. Every day you must ask whether your body is as fully coordinated as it is supposed to be.

What can you do to bring your body into coordination with the divine blueprint that you wrote and that is stored in your etheric placenta? Below is an exercise to help you fine-tune the vibrations of your body. Your body will then become more alert and impart its wisdom on a feeling level for all the answers you seek in all your experiences. Innermost divine guidance becomes part of your life. When you are in rhythm with and attuned to your body, it will inspire you to coordinate with other levels of reality and other humans on the physical plane. We encourage you to frequently undertake this exercise. It will balance your life.

There are energies going from the back of your ears into your kidneys and your second chakra. These energies bring understanding for the karmic experience you must balance. Since you do not remember these experiences, this energy affects your second chakra, and you take actions from there.

When you are in coordination with your body, you become aware of this energy and take action. This energy attracts situations and experiences through which you can heal your karma. Your actions are then motivated by your desire to complete the energies you have come here to master, not by a fear about survival.

Do Not Run

Energies also flow up from the soles of your feet to your knees. There are chakras in the back of your knees, and when you attune to them, they help you remember the purpose for which you were born.

When you look at the deepest level, you can see that most people run from life because they fear it. By becoming aware of the energy rising from your feet to your knees, you will understand that you have the capacity to do what you came here to do, and you will also remember that you cannot run. You have to stay here to complete what you have come here to complete. When you do not complete these lessons, you come back again and again until you do. Imagine how many soul promises you have made to yourself that you did not complete in other lifetimes. It is cumulative. You come back again and again to try to fulfill them.

I ask you to embrace the wisdom that running will not solve your problems. Running will chase you all the way to hell (if you believe in a hell). It is very important that you start feeling the confidence to face everything in your life. The energy to do this is in the back of your knees.

Connect with Your I Am Presence through Your Thumbs

Now I will show you where you can feel the energy that connects you with other humans and other realities: It is in the thumbs. When you connect with your thumbs regularly, your intuitive inspiration flows more readily and you become an excellent channel. Archangel Gabriel has told you that your thumb represents the Christ consciousness, or the God presence within you [See *Dance of the Hands*, Light Technology Publishing, 2015].

Close your eyes and ask one thumb to give you a message. Allow this to happen. When you connect with this energy, you remember what you have come here to do and know you have the ability to do it. You see incredible light pour out of your thumbs and become a huge fountain of light, and you are inside it.

✳   ✳   ✳

I am Archangel Michael. The thumb represents the Christ consciousness and holds the Metatronic energies. If you work with your thumbs, they will become very powerful healing tools. You can press your thumbs on certain parts of a body, and healing will occur. You can also remember your star heritage by working with your thumbs. Press both thumbs together in front of your heart and chant "so" three times. [Chants: So, so, so.] You will feel very grounded, and you will become certain of the message you receive. This will immediately give you a sense of confidence.

Sacred Travel

There is an angel of travel. When you are ready to incarnate as part of your soul's blueprint, you make a plan to travel during your life. You choose the places to visit in a lifetime based on what you want to learn and remember. You might have had past karmic relationships somewhere, and you'd like to go back to heal them. You might go to other places to collect energy to help you remember.

Most people do not ask their souls whether travel is appropriate or part of their souls' blueprint. People allow their minds to decide where they travel, or they are inspired to go somewhere their friends have gone. There is nothing wrong with that. There is beauty and growth in those experiences as well. However, when you travel to destinations you chose before you were born, you advance your spiritual growth and fulfill your life contacts. For example, your might have set up a contract to walk the Andalusian trails to heal your karma and enhance your spiritual growth. There are lines on the soles of your feet that reveal the travel energy of your life.

❋　❋　❋

Soul Journeys

Blessings. We are called Hritorhm. We are the angels of sacred travel, and we support the understanding and remembrance of your energetic connection to places where you have planned to travel. We have never spoken to human beings before. It is an honor to be able to speak with you.

Do you know that you travel when you sleep? You can program your sleep travel to destinations you want to visit and still be aware of them consciously. Some of the contracts you have made are not only for places on Earth but also for systems in other galaxies. This is called soul travel, and it will help you understand many things.

We encourage you to take soul journeys. If you cannot travel physically on the Earth plane, then you can make a soul journey as part of your soul blueprint. If you have forgotten your blueprint, meditate on the places you have made contracts to visit. All humans have at least five to seven places they need to visit as part of their soul blueprints to help them awaken. If you cannot go somewhere physically, use soul travel. You will fulfill your soul contract, and this will help you remember.

You have also made contracts to take soul journeys to the animal kingdom. Ask for these contracts to be activated and released so that you can understand them. Animals hold certain vibrational frequencies. If animals were not on the planet, human life expectancy would be very short, fewer than fifty years. Animals have a very important role to play in human life because people have a deep karmic connection with them. Animals carry certain frequencies and qualities that you can use for enhancement. The great shamans do this by becoming deer, gorillas, bison, polar bears, or cheetahs. Ask if part of your soul journey contract is with the animal kingdom.

You can travel to the crystal kingdom as well. When you connect with the beings of the crystal kingdom, you clearly remember your role in Atlantis, what you did there, and what you are here to do.

When you take these journeys, you will not only enjoy them but also notice growth in your perceptions. After you become proficient at this, you may wish to take a soul journey to the heart of the Creator. A beautiful golden boat will appear in front of you. Sit in this golden boat, and travel up and up and up into the light. Then submerge in the light. Blessings, we are the angel of travel, Hritorhm.

※　　※　　※

This is Archangel Michael. Would anyone like to ask a question?

Is "soul travel" another term for bilocation or astral projection?

Soul travel is done in your physical body. You become aware of it, and you return with energy and information about what you saw and gained. It is more than astral projection. Bilocation is a little bit different. Bilocation is being in two or more places at the same time while you remain at home. Soul travel is a spiritual journey but in a physical body. You leave, but you become aware that your body remains. You go to other realities and return with a full understanding and remembrance of what happened in those realities.

We hope you enjoyed the little chat with this beautiful angel, for this angel also supports ascended masters. One of you may want to take a journey to my ashram on the crystal mountain, where many ascended masters gather and refresh themselves. Blessings.

Use Your Name to Attract What You Want in Life

We extend our deepest love and gratitude to the brothers and sisters of light who participate from all countries. When we have these sessions, we do not just talk to people; we set up a light grid. Just imagine how much power it holds and how much energy is downloaded into Earth. You can bring in higher vibrations because when the grid becomes stronger, more and more light comes through. In recent months, the messages coming through have been much deeper than in past work. You are strengthening the grid. Your grid is tremendously affecting the planet, so we thank you for this.

Now we would like to bring forward the angel of names. The vibrations you hold are in your name, your life path, your challenges, and your karmic contracts. There are angels who work with names, and we are honored that this angel speaks.

✳   ✳   ✳

Hello, friends, my name is Nehur-Ra-Sim. I am called on to work with the benevolent energies that are encoded in names and can be of benefit.

Each of you carries individual life contracts and life paths. Some people have contracts to be teachers, some are in other service-related sectors, and some are simply to be who they are, holding the vibration and frequency to help with transitions.

Everything in the universe has a name, including the Creator (who is called by many names). All angels have names. All stars have names. All guides have names. These names crisscross, sending out energy and drawing forth what is needed. You can use names to call forth exactly what you want in life. Here is an example: Let's say your name is Atchison. You can use the vibration of the letter N to go forth and bring you the result you seek. Other people who have the letter N in their names will respond to you much faster because you carry a similar vibration and will draw each other forth. This is the power of attraction.

Life partners and business partners have many similar letters in their names, bringing the gifts of understanding, appreciating life paths and plans, and recognizing solutions. We encourage you to look at this. You can write down all the things you want to achieve in your life and use the frequencies of your name to attract what you want. You might say that sounds too simple. Yes, it is simple. That is the beauty of it. This understanding has not been given before.

Write the letters of your name on a piece of paper. Next, ask for what you are trying to achieve and how you can use your name to attract it. Then pick one letter. For example, let's say your name is Robert and you select the letter R. Call forth people who can support you in your project (or something you want to create). There is a high likelihood that you will meet people who also have that letter in their names. When that happens, you will know that you are in the flow of things and everything will work out. If you attract a person who has two Rs in his or her name, take note because this is definitely a sign from the universe!

We encourage you to work with this. Through using your name, you can shift many areas of your life. Each letter in your name carries vibrational frequencies that match your karmic contract. When you use your name, you call forth people who are part of your karmic life contract and life lessons. You want to call forth only benevolent experiences. You must say, "I use my name to call forth people who will support me in what I am trying to solve, answer, or create." You will be amazed. We encourage you to look into this. Now I'm open to questions.

Does it matter which letter we choose?

No. Write down what you want to achieve, then meditate, and ask which letter in your name you should use.

If I were to use the first letter of my name, am I inviting the energy and everything that starts with that letter?

Exactly. You will see how powerful you are — how powerful human beings are — by using your name. You can use your name to draw forth what you want, and you will complete your life path. Sometimes your life path is not simply about challenges. Karmic contracts are not merely about challenges. Karmic contracts can also imply that you break through and claim certain things. Many life lessons are about being successful, breaking through patterns and behaviors, and claiming your true power. It is a challenge to break through and claim your magnificence in every area.

My name is not my birth name. This is the name given through marriage.

Use the name you presently have and use frequently. You will use your name as an antenna to draw forth what you want.

✳   ✳   ✳

This is Archangel Michael. When you get the hang of how to work with the letters of your name, you might want to work with star systems using the letters of their names. If you know the names of the star systems, you can bring about incredible energy, and there will be a shift. Through the law of attraction, when you send out an inspirational energy, the resonance creates a response that has a similar vibrational energy. Stars are looking to make a connection with you. They might not know you personally, but they are looking to make connections with people who have similar vibrational frequencies. You are beaming light, and they are beaming light. *Boom!* A joining can happen.

Every letter can be used to attract what you want in life, but certain letters have more power and meaning. One is Z. One is K. One is P. One is S. Another is A. Look into these. At first, write down what you want to create, and work with a letter in your name to attract what you want. Once you get used to that, you can go into more complex things. This will expand your capacity to think of higher and bigger things, solve problems, attract what you seek, and create the highest good for you and everybody else. Be aware that this works both positively and negatively, so you must always say, "I am using my name to draw forth only positive, benevolent, loving experiences." Blessings.

Understand Your Life Path

We have another angel to speak with you. This angel holds the energy and the frequency to understand your life path. The ascended masters and your guides help you, but they do not clearly tell you about your life path. They help you see the hints, for hints show you the direction. If you are aware, then you come to know. If you want to clearly understand your life path, then call on the Angel Sadha.

✳   ✳   ✳

Hello, blessed ones. We are Sadha, the angels supporting you in redis-covering your life path. Human beings have asked three questions from time immemorial: "Who am I?" "Where am I from?" and "What is my purpose?" There is a blueprint for your life and your life path on each life stream on this and other planets and in other stars systems. It is encoded in different times and different realities. Your blueprint is also encoded in the heart and solar plexus of Mother Earth and in certain life forms, such as giant trees, whales, and deer. These beings are here for only one reason: to help you unravel your blueprint, for there are certain animal energies coming into your solar plexus. There is a push-pull of energy in your solar plexus. Animals can only send energy to you, but it is up to you to receive it. At the deepest level, you want to open these energies, but your mind does not understand. Subconsciously you want to open it, but you do not know how.

We encourage you to call on these animal beings. Many people think the blueprint is in the third eye. The original energy of your blueprint is in your solar plexus. We ask you to focus there and raise the energy into your third eye by using these animals. You will then be able to understand your blueprint and your life path through your third eye. It will become an experiential understanding.

To become aware of your solar plexus, point the index, middle, and ring fingers of your right hand toward the area between your second and third chakras. Hold these fingers two or three inches in front of this area, making slow clockwise circles (you are facing the clock). You will feel energy in your spinal column.

When you feel energy and warmth there, push it out through your third eye. You will immediately feel a sense of warm energy coming out. It will flow into your hands. Extend your palms, and say, "I send this energy into my auric body." Your auric body also contains your blueprint. Then say, "I send this energy to the spinal column of Mother Earth and into the trees, the whales, and the deer."

In a matter of days, you will feel the energy of your life path. You may have visions, inspiration, dreams, serendipity, or coincidence guiding you to your true path of why you are here. A sense of knowingness will come to you. Everything in your body will speak and work to hold your blue-print, releasing its core energy into you, and you will surely know. You will never have to ask; you will know.

Activate the Sacred Fire

Close your eyes. Call on us, Sadha. See three beings of light standing around you: one at the back of your head and one on either side. The angel at the back of your head places her hand on your back, on your ascension chakra [above the medulla]. The other two angels place their hands on your temples, sending light into them. You will see a sacred triangular energy form shooting up through the middle of your head, and a sacred fire will begin to burn.

Ask the sacred fire to descend slowly into your solar plexus. The sacred fire has a sound frequency. As it slowly descends, you will hear its sound. Allow the sacred fire to emanate from your solar plexus.

See the sacred fire become three fires, one extending from your solar plexus, one in front of you, and one twirling behind you in your spinal column. The sacred fire in your solar plexus moves to the top of your head. The three sacred fires are connected, and a triangle forms. See the sacred fires become three more sacred fires above you. You now have three fires above and three fires below. See these merge as a star, and you are inside it. You are the star of light, the star of fire. See the star turn into a circle, and the circle is around you, the sacred circle of fire.

Say these words three times: "El Shadai. El Shadai. El Shadai." Make the statement, "I anchor this sacred circle of fire around me eternally, and I exist in it from now on, for I am the fire, I am the light, and I am God."

After you complete this, breathe deeply three times, and send this high frequency of energy into the ground. Gently open your eyes.

* * *

I am Archangel Michael. This magical fire exists in all hearts and endures whether a being is living or dead. When you die, this fire is not activated. It goes back into its original form but still remains as a point of energy. This is the fire that Metatron talks about, the fire in which you are not consumed but are healed completely.

This circle of fire stays with you every day. You carry it within you. It will make you feel vigorous and enthusiastic because it is the life force coming into you. You will gain a thirst for life, and you will become passionate, intuitive, and creative. You will see every moment as sacred and holy. When someone appears in your life, you might or might not help that person, but you will know he or she came to give you a gift. This person appears in your life to receive a gift from you just as you receive a gift from him or her. Let's suppose you encounter a homeless person. You might give that person money, but what gift did he or she give you? He gave you the opportunity to experience wholeness within yourself, the opportunity to express your sacredness. It works two ways. Blessings.

※　　※　　※

Hello, I am Elijah. I am not part of the angelic realm, but I suggest you remember one thing: What you do has an effect on the planet. Hold this thought in your heart. It is not wasting time. You are building energies, bridges of light among people and countries, and this light even goes into other realms and realities. Many in the astral realm will benefit from the light you create so that they can return and find the love of God in their hearts. The sacred fire given here is the sacred fire through which you gain your inner connection. When you meditate with the sacred circle of fire, you will see it slowly expand and multiply. It will become six sacred circles of fire. Through this fire, one is liberated. Blessings.

※　　※　　※

Heal Timelines and Create an Optimum Future

Blessed ones, we carry the imprint and the energy of the one you call Scargohsa, and we heal past timelines and draw future timelines into your present reality. This is an important time in your planet's history. You are now able to understand the influence of the past and how your future is determined, how a planet's future is made, and how Earth people's consciousness as a whole is made. Much of this is about past timelines. You know that the past determines the present and the present determines the future.

On the timeline, look at when this planet was created. Your planet is almost 4.5 billion years old. There were times when this planet was mined by extraterrestrial beings for its precious minerals. Even as recently as ten years ago, extraterrestrials attempted to mine these precious metals. This affects the consciousness of the planet.

Since the industrial revolution, Earth's resources have been greatly misused. When the earth is damaged, people's consciousnesses are also damaged. Oil is a gift from Mother Earth, but it should be extracted and used in a most sacred way. However, it has been used for different purposes and extracted with greed and without a spiritual context. Uranium is the brain of Mother Earth. When uranium is taken from Earth, it is as if someone removed part of her brain. Would you be able to think clearly if that happened to you?

When materials are taken from Mother Earth's body, it affects her consciousness. There has been a breakage in the consciousness of Mother Earth. Many benevolent timelines would have happened but for the uncaring way natural resources have been taken from the ground. The energy of benevolent timelines is anchored in the ground, and when the earth is disturbed, that energy is cut and the timeline does not flow. This timeline would have created a new future for humanity and Mother Earth. Many such breakages have affected human consciousness.

When human beings were created as God humans (Adam Kadmon), a seed atom was placed in the core of each being, and this atom was supposed to blossom to its full potential. Because of mining, that timeline did not happen. Since you are part of Mother Earth's body, that affected your consciousness and your personal time and reality. There are exercises that can heal Mother Earth's timeline. This directly corresponds with your timeline, for Mother Earth holds a blueprint of your perfection.

Your soul group is held by five energetic configurations. One is under the sphinx. Another is held by Mother Earth herself. When she is disturbed and that timeline is lost, your timeline is also damaged. Many ancient shamans understood this concept, and they had ceremonies to realign Mother Earth to reestablish the benevolent timeline so that human beings could reinstate their own benevolent timelines.

The future of humanity is simple. It is not only to ascend but also to become the main consciousness for a developing planet. That planet is being created right now. The predominant consciousness of that planet will be the new consciousness of humanity. If your consciousness is high enough and you are all able to ascend in 300 years, then the ascension energy of your whole planet will incorporate into the new planet. The new beings who will live on that planet will begin as ascended beings. This is why it is very important to work with timelines and bring healing. You become a part of the cocreative process with the Creator in developing a new consciousness for the new planet.

This new planet will come into force in about 2,000 years. It is still being made. A planet requires much work, and 2,000 years is a very short time. By that time, Earth will have ascended. Every human being will have had a golden era of peace. The consciousness from this planet will be shared, and that will be the predominant consciousness in the new planet. That is the destiny for human beings.

How can you heal the past timelines so that you can heal the present and move into the future? Hypnotherapists can access memories of what happened in the past to help cure phobias, limitations, and blockages. One timeline might have a strong impact on a person's reality. This is a noble process, but few people can access this information and use it to create new timelines. They must have some spiritual understanding of reincarnation that they bring from other timelines.

Anchor a Fifth-Dimensional Timeline to Your Third-Dimensional Body

You are tied to your personal timeline for your evolution in the back of your shoulders. Bring your attention to the back of your shoulders, and bring your scapulas together. That is where your personal timelines are anchored. Mother Earth's timeline is anchored to the backs of your knees. There is a strong correlation between the shoulders and the knees. Focus on your scapulas and the backs of the knees.

See a stream of light pouring from the left scapula to the back of your left knee and likewise on the right side. Visualize two tubes of light flowing from top to bottom and back again. Visualize a circle in the back of your body that is connected to these two tubes of light. See a golden pot inside the circle with a sacred fire burning in it. Ask that all distorted energy from the broken timeline be brought into the sacred fire to be transmuted. You might feel some sensations (even some sadness) or see some images, especially of darkness or fear. Allow anything to surface. If you see an initial image, a thought process, or a feeling, visualize them as going into the fire in the golden pot and burning and transmuting. Allow this to happen.

Say, "All the timelines that were distorted in my personal reality from the time of Adam Kadmon to now are transmuting in this flame." Breathe.

Now I, Angel Scargohsa, step behind you and place my hands on your scapulas. I transmit energy and implant a sacred code — a sacred geometric pattern, a triangle of energy — that goes all the way to your hips. It is a golden triangle. In the middle of the triangle, I place a golden sphere. The top of the sphere is about two inches above the golden triangle, touching your medulla oblongata, where your ascension chakra is located. There is energy in this golden triangle and in the sphere. The sphere touches your head, opening an eleven-point star. This is the ascension chakra star.

You can see the eleven-point star slowly open and pulse with a silver-white light combined with soft purple and magenta. The light from the ascension chakra flows into the triangle; from the triangle, it flows into the circle; and from the circle, it flows into the two tubes of light running from your scapulas to the backs of your knees.

A beautiful silver, soft-purple, and magenta light fills your entire being and surrounds you. You are now inside this light. Allow for this to happen. A merkabah appears. Step into it, for it is your personal vehicle. It is your carriage. Envision it taking off. It goes to Arcturus, to the ascension portal for human beings and the temple of ascension, where your fifth-dimensional lightbody now exists. This is your perfect body. See this perfect being come toward you. Look into its eyes. Embrace this being, and see yourself merge with it. Breathe it in, and say, "Ina, I am. Ina, I am. Ina, I am." You have become one with the being. Breathe. Allow this energy to flow through your being. Visualize your entire body fill with the light from your perfected self.

Ask that any blockages you still have in your physical body open up and release. Visualize every meridian in your body fill with the light of your fifth-dimensional, perfect self. Say, "All past timelines are dissolved in the light of my perfected self." Allow for this.

Ask a question about any area of your life. For example, ask, "What is my future potential in the timeline of 2018 for relationships, health, work, or abundance?" When you see what you like, breathe into it.

Since you now hold fifth-dimensional energy, you will draw that energy to you by the intention of your thought. Breathe into that. See this energy go into your third-dimensional body, which has merged with your fifth-dimensional energy in the timeline between your shoulders and the backs of your knees. Breathe, and see the new timeline become stronger as an energy embedded in your knees and shoulders.

Open your palms, and breathe energy into the past. You might feel a tingling sensation. When you feel energy in your palms, bring it into your solar plexus. Bring both palms to your solar plexus, and anchor the energy there.

Say, "I pass this energy into the point of power within me, for this is my new timeline, and I am drawing this new timeline into my present reality."

See this energy become stronger in your solar plexus. Breathe it in. Breathe it in. See it become solid in your solar plexus. Release your palms. Breathe. Breathe once again.

Dear ones, you have brought forth a future timeline and anchored it into your point of power in your solar plexus. Every time you think about the new timeline, send energy into your solar plexus. All this energy exists there.

In the next several days, beam energy there. You will see that what you draw forth will become clearer in your life, and the manifestation will happen more quickly. Some of you will be able to manifest what you see for 2018 in the next four months. You will see the effect of this in your life during the next four months if you work at this every day.

Blessings. I am the angel Scargohsa with Archangel Michael. I will take questions.

If we do this, how will it affect other people? Will it affect their free will?

No. You are working from a higher reality. Creating what is best for you will not infringe on the free will of others. Your focus should be on you — what is the highest and most beneficial for you. When you create what is benevolent for you, others will naturally be uplifted by your creation.

This felt like housecleaning.

Exactly, but in a much greater way. It is a complete renovation of the house. We are giving you tools and initiating you into a new reality. One of the realities in the new consciousness is that you must trust in the unseen and have faith that when you make an intention, the energy will appear in your energy field.

❋　❋　❋

Attract Nine Significant People to Your Life

This is Archangel Michael. We would like to bring an angel who can help you attract benevolent and helpful people to your life. You have heard the expression, "No man is an island." You grow through other people.

Everything that happens in your life — whether positive, loving, or something else — happens through other people, for they bring you growth. You call them forth to bring you an experience so that you can express who you are during that experience, and through that experience, you realize who you are, and you grow. There are supporting energies such as angels who you can call to speed the process of drawing people into your life to support you in creating a new timeline or reality. One of the angels you can work with is Citrayomhei. Let us invite this angel to speak.

✳   ✳   ✳

Blessings to my dear family of the Earth plane. This is Citrayomhei: It is always a joy to bring our understanding and to connect with the beautiful people of Earth. You were in a unique experiment, and you have successfully emerged from it. You are seeing the aftereffects, the last part of a cleansing process. You passed the test. The planet is intact and will not be destroyed, no matter who says what. There will be channelings about what will happen — people beaming off the planet and some left behind. Nothing of this sort will happen. This was a test, and you passed it. We will assist others when they pass it. All of you are becoming elders. We ask you to hold that title in your hearts, for you will lead others in their completion processes.

Each of you on Earth has nine people in your life who play significant roles. These nine people are there to create good times and good experiences for you. You can call these nine people forth. You might already have some of them in your life. Some might say they are not spiritual. They might lead you to your path and then move away. However, they often become your friends for life, always supporting and loving you. These people will touch you deeply. They are part of your soul contract and part of the supporting energies you brought with you. They might be teachers, coworkers, or people you shared much of your life with or who even changed your life completely. They are rarely family members. These nine will often enlighten you, take you to your ascension path, and help you with your ascension. They will usually be on their own paths of self-awareness and self-discovery. The ninth person will almost certainly be the person who leads your ascension. All the others will help you navigate this lifetime, creating benevolent, loving experiences. They will support you and love you for who you are.

The energy of the significant nine people is in the middle of your forehead, just above the angel chakra [at the hairline]. Bring your attention to about an inch above your angel chakra, about two inches above your third eye. This is the place where you hold energy for the nine people who can come into your life to support your soul growth and help you find your soul's path.

Visualize a circle. The circle is divided into quarters. Working counter-clockwise from the upper-left quadrant in the first quarter, you see the numbers 1 and 2, and beneath that, you see the numbers 3, 4, and 5. In the lower right quadrant, you see 6, 7, and 8, and in the quadrant above that, 9.

Focus on the 9, and see the circle on your forehead start to spin. See the circle move backward into your head, your brain, your ears, your hands, your feet, and Earth.

See a stream of golden energy flow from your toes and become a small pathway. From now on, every time you take a step on the ground, this golden consciousness will go out from your feet into the land and will spread into the ground. It will touch those nine people, and they will start to appear in your life. We cannot say when they will appear or what they will look like, but if you work with this, you will likely meet two or three of them before the end of the year. Just breathe in, and anchor this golden light into the ground.

Every day when you step out of the house, visualize the golden light from your feet going into the ground and spreading through it. People who are part of your soul contract will feel the vibration of the golden light coming from you, and they will be drawn into your life, sometimes through accidents, sometimes through introductions, and sometimes through chance meetings. You will feel as if a connection can happen, for these people are part of the support group you brought into your life when you were born. It is very simple and effective.

* * *

Does a person's age determine how many of these people he or she might have already met?
This is Archangel Michael. There might be more than nine significant people in someone's life, but certainly nine will have a very big effect. Sometimes they can deeply touch your life. You will not stay with

them all the time, but they will have a big effect that influences many areas of your life. These nine people will be wonderful and will only create positive, loving experiences in your life. These are people who are only here to support and love you. You will know, in an instant, through your heart.

CHAPTER SEVEN

Clear Karmic Energy

Angel Barbiel, Angel Zahariel, Angel Ginaomayar, Angel Samshie,
Creator, Angel Beihiyud, Archangel Michael, and Angel Esausraham

Hello, blessed ones. My name is Barbiel. We are the angels of feeling good about yourself. Feeling good is very important. You must feel good about yourself. You might call it self-esteem or joy to love yourself. It is very difficult for human beings to love themselves because they lack self-esteem. You begin a lifetime with karma and life lessons, and self-esteem is basic to working through both of these. If you have self-esteem, you believe in yourself and can overcome all karmic challenges and learn the lessons you have come here to master. Self-esteem is the key to human liberation. People who believe in themselves make a difference to this planet. Their self-esteem does not come from foolishness or ego; it comes from understanding their self-worth and their purpose for being here.

Consider Mahatma Gandhi. In spite of great obstacles, he believed in himself completely, and he liberated millions of people. Self-esteem is critical. Napoleon Bonaparte believed in himself and had clothes made so that he could dress like a commander-in-chief. He visualized, practiced, and believed in himself completely. When you have self-esteem and believe in yourself, you are courageous and never defeated, no matter what. At times, you might feel despair and take a rest, but you never give up.

All people who have made positive contributions to the world have had very high self-esteem. Explorers who went to the Arctic, who crossed the great oceans on voyages of discovery, or who flew a solar-powered airplane across the Atlantic overcame the limitations they came here to conquer and made history.

Boost Your Self-Esteem

How can you have self-esteem when you came here with self-created limitations? Although your base chakra holds the limitations and the energies of survival and poverty consciousness, the other side of the coin is that you also carry the energies of self-esteem.

Close your eyes. Bring your attention to your base chakra, and breathe from there. See a beautiful gold coin there with an emblem embedded on each side. One side has the image of a crab, representing limitations. A crab will always pull at the other crabs trying to climb out of the bucket. It represents the human mind and belief systems that try to pull you down by saying such things as, "It is not possible. I am not ready. I do not know how to do it. I am not fortunate enough. I have tried so many things that have not worked. I am a failure. I was not born with a silver spoon in my mouth. I had to struggle to pay the bills," and on and on and on. The other side of the coin has a beautiful butterfly. On the coin embedded in your base chakra, the butterfly faces upward, and the crab faces downward.

Visualize energy from the butterfly flowing up through your chakra column and your crown chakra and falling around you like a shower of light. See the energy from the crab going downward through the soles of your feet into the ground, where it is transmuted and goes into Mother Earth's body as a healing light.

* * *

Rise above the Drudgery

Hello, my friends and family. My name is Zahariel. I am the angel of enthusiasm, cheerfulness, brightness, and vigor. These are qualities of God. How many human beings live with these qualities? Very few. For most people, life is drudgery. There is no excitement or passion. They go on living and thinking this is reality. It is the reality they have created. No matter how difficult their circumstances are, there are still pockets of time when they could incorporate these qualities in their lives. This is one of the life lessons for human beings. Despite the challenges, can you still find joy and peace? You could say that life is very difficult. We understand.

Can someone who lives in a war zone in Afghanistan or a mother with starving children find some joy and peace despite the circumstances?

We say yes, but on a very high spiritual level. This is one lesson. These people have come to learn from these experiences. We help them when we can. Remember that their circumstances were chosen by their souls to create experiences through which they could learn.

Consider a mother with starving children in Syria. What can she do? Despite her circumstances, could she find a moment to appreciate what she has in her life rather than focusing on what she does not have? This is very difficult to practice. If she were to do that — focus on the bright, cheerful aspects of her life and on the light — even for the shortest period, she could shift her condition immediately. Her soul is trying to teach her this.

When you experience difficult times, look at things from a different angle and realize that all your attention is focused on the challenges. Are there other areas of your life in which you can find a moment for cheerfulness? When you look at your life, you can see there are always other areas you can focus on. When you focus on cheerful aspects, enthusiasm comes forward and dissolves your problems.

All of you are lightworkers. You have high frequencies of light, and the energy you hold will expand. That energy will take over and completely defuse difficult situations. This is not easy to practice because you have been conditioned to believe that your inner experiences are tied to your outer experiences. You connect your inner peace with your outer experiences.

Come to a middle ground to see your circumstances from a larger perspective. For at least five minutes a day, hold that cheerfulness as truth. After you visualize it, you will see a shift. Your soul will shift that experience because you understood the lesson.

Burn Karmic Energies

There are balls of energy beneath your toes. When you wake in the morning, close your eyes, and bring your attention to all your toes. Spread them as wide as you can, and breathe through them. Breathe through the center of your toes. Breathe it in.

Visualize breathing in a bright metallic yellow through the soles of your feet. Bring this yellow light up to your ankles and through your thighs, and anchor it into your base chakra. Once again, breathe through the toes and then go up. Anchor the light into your base chakra. One more time: breathe, and then let it go.

Visualize the bright yellow mixing with the red of the base chakra. A flame appears in your base chakra. See it shoot up like a beam of light. Let it shoot above your head and into your soul star chakra. It will go up into the tenth chakra. This is about one arm's length above your head. See this beam of light go down through the pranic tube, which is like a huge pillar of light, into the back of your body and down to your toes.

Again, take this light through your toes to the base chakra. Bright yellow mixes with a beautiful red, and a flame appears. The flame shoots up all the way to the tenth chakra that is one arm's length above your head. A tube runs parallel to the back of your body, and the flame goes downward into this tube and deep into the ground. Then it comes back to your toes.

Breathe this for a few minutes. Breathe it in. Breathe it in. Breathe it in. Continue breathing this beautiful light, circulating it from your toes and bringing it to the back of your body.

See this light settling into your hips. Let the flame burn brightly there. Breathe into this flame. This flame has the capacity to burn through many karmic energies stored in the back of your body. The situation you are in and the challenges you experience result from your karmic energy and the life lessons you chose to bring in. This flame has the capacity to burn through much of that.

Feel the heat of the flame. Breathe it in. See the flame shoot through the back of your body and up through the back of the neck into your ascension chakra [at the back of your head]. Bring it to the top of your head, and anchor it into your crown chakra. See your crown chakra explode with streams of colored light that go all the way up to the tenth chakra and shower around you. You are bathed in these colors. Allow for the explosion of light to flow through your crown area and fall around you. Breathe. Breathe. Breathe. Let it go deep into the ground, into the bosom of Mother Earth. When you are cheerful, bright, and enthusiastic, Mother Earth also is healed. Let us go deep into the ground and anchor into it.

We ask you to do this exercise once a day for several days. It will become part of your energy field. This practice will help you find pockets of tranquility, peace, joy, and appreciation for life. Your focus on problems shifts slightly, even if only for a brief time, such as a half-hour. That half-hour can cause a shift in the energy field around you. This energy, the energy of God, is a high frequency. Blessings, blessings, blessings. We are the Angel Zahariel, angel of brightness, enthusiasm, and cheerfulness.

✳ ✳ ✳

Clear Behavior and Thought Patterns from Family Lineage

Blessings, dear family, this is Ginaomayar, and I heal the patterns, behaviors, thought forms, and sicknesses you brought through your genetic lineage. We are not from this universe. Did you know there is a planet of angels? It is in a different universe. Archangel Michael asked me to share my light, wisdom, and love with all of you, for you are teachers in training. You have the potential to start teaching in the next several months. You will teach about how you found your ascension path in your own way, what the pitfalls were, and how you maneuvered through them. When you teach, you also learn and grow.

You carry many patterns and behaviors from your parents and grandparents — your family lineage — and the cultural lineage of your country. Before you were born, your soul had meetings to make your blueprint and to plan the things you would do, the parents you would have, the type of body you would inhabit, and your inclinations and limitations. During these soul meetings, the higher selves of your relatives and parents were present to set up the limitations of old behaviors that come from your family lineage. Your parents and your family do this in service so that you could break out of these patterns and heal them. You heal these patterns not only for yourself but also for them. They were not aware of these patterns when they were alive on the planet. When they passed away, they could see these energies. This is why they met with you to make your blueprint. They asked you to break these patterns to set them free.

Defuse the Energies of Your Family Lineage

The energies of your family lineage are stored above your solar plexus and go to the back of your body. *Visualize a triangle above your solar plexus. This triangle is so embedded in your solar plexus that you can see it from the back of your body. In this triangle, see a soft-beige liquid energy. This liquid energy contains the energies of past patterns, behaviors, and thought forms. They were deliberately placed there for you to overcome them. Breathe in the liquid energy. Breathe. See the liquid inside the triangle turn to vapor. Breathe. Send energy there to become vaporous. It pushes out. All the vapor goes into the ether and converts to golden consciousness.*

The triangle above your solar plexus now is empty. See a golden spirit there, filling up the triangle. Open your palms, and ask the energy from this triangle to come into both hands. See flames coming from both hands. Combine your hands to make one flame. Bring your hands to your heart, and say, "I bring the healing light of the golden one into myself, releasing all the old patterns of genetic imprints, especially regarding thought patterns and behaviors. I release all geometric patterns these created that are not in harmony with my original blueprint."

See the golden triangle above your solar plexus again. See a golden circle with twelve spokes that spins inside the triangle. It rotates and grows larger and larger, creating a mandala. The mandala becomes bigger than you, and soon you are inside the mandala. Breathe it in. Say, "I am one with this new creation, this new mandala of me." You become the mandala.

This is your chakra mandala, the all enlightening and fulfilling mandala. This is the key to manifesting your new reality because when you heal your genetic lineage, you unleash incredible amounts of light and release false belief systems. You have faith in yourself and trust yourself. You have self-confidence, and you love yourself. You are the mandala. Breathe it in. Breathe it in. Breathe it in.

The great teacher Sanat Kumara steps forward and places his ascension wand on your third eye, sending a beam of light into the mandala you have become. It fills the mandala with ever-growing light. You are the light. You are no longer a body. You are no longer a mind. You are no longer a soul. You are light.

See only one light, a flame burning. There is nothing else. This is you, a beautiful lamp. You have become unburdened by the lineage of family thinking, thought patterns, and behaviors, particularly the limitations of such false thoughts and belief systems as, "You cannot do this," "you are not good enough to do this," or "you can never achieve this." Let them go.

When in doubt, visualize the lamp and light in the exercise, and focus on the sacred geometry of your solar plexus, the triangle with the spokes in a circle. Breathe, and let it become your chakra mandala every time you are in fear. Let it enfold you, and you will immediately come back into your new reality. Breathe. Say, "I give intention to hold this frequency, this light, within every cell of my body. Every cell is filled with incredible light, for I am the light. I am the light. I am the light."

This is angel Ginaomayar. My love is always with you. You can call on me anytime, and I will embrace you in the fold of my wings. Blessings. Are there questions?

I have a lot of my mother in me. I feel it. I act like her. When I feel this, can I call on you to help me change that vibration and that pattern?

Of course. Also call Archangel Gabriel, the angel of the morning sun.

✳ ✳ ✳

Use Water to Clear and Expand Your Consciousness

Hello, my dear friends. My name is Samshie. I am one of the angels who support water and water beings. Water is a very sacred part of life. You can live without food, but you cannot live without water. Much has been written about water, and I would like to briefly touch on some important aspects that haven't been discussed.

There are energies beneath your fingernails. Have you ever wondered why nails grow? Your nails hold memories. You shed something when nails grow and are cut. But there are certain frequencies of light energy beneath the nails called etheric healing chakras, and you can use water to activate them.

Fill a bowl with water, and dip your fingertips in it. Close your eyes, and bring your attention to the fingertips of both hands and make this sound: "Shaaam, shaaam." Repeat it nine times. This activates healing energy beneath your nails. It flows backward through the backs of your wrists to the chakras on your shoulders, alpha and omega. These two chakras are the chakras for karma. By doing this, you release and erase many karmic energies that are already finished in this timeline. You decommission and deactivate dormant karmic energies in your physical body.

Make this energy flow into the back of your body, into your hips, into your feet, into the ground, and back to the elements once again. You will feel a sense of lightness.

You can also activate the Christ consciousness with water. *Wet your hands. Close your eyes, and bring your attention to your thumbs. Close your hands to make fists. Relax your fists, and let your thumbs stand up. There are miniature sacred geometric patterns in your thumbs. Bring your attention to your thumbs, and ask that the eight sacred geometrical patterns there be activated. Say, "I ask the eight octaves of healing to take place through the underworld and the overworld, and I give the intention to activate the Christ consciousness within me now." If your thumbs are wet, you will feel powerful energy.*

Allow the energy to flow from your thumbs into your hand and throughout your physical body. You will feel pulsing light within and throughout your body.

Create the web of the golden one with water by putting your feet in a big bowl that has enough water in it to cover your ankles. Visualize breathing the water through your feet, in and out through your feet. You feel incredible light energies — light particles — come into you, making an oval shape around your ankles. You feel lightness and a lessening of the magnetics in your physical body. This light moves upward and settles in your solar plexus, creating a web of light there and throughout your body. This web grows very large, and you are in the middle, like a spider.

This is called the web of the golden one. When you are in it, your circular wisdom will be fully opened [See *DNA of the Spirit, Volume 1,* Light Technology Publishing: 2014, p. 297 for an explanation of circular wisdom]. You are one with the web of life, the web of the universe, and it will expand with each breath. The stars are connected to this web of light.

Your web of light extends to other webs of light. This means your soul extends into other souls. There is no longer separation between you and other human beings. You are all part of one web of light.

Good day to you. I am the angel of water, Samshie. We will have more to say. Today we just want to give you a taste of what we are here to teach you. Blessings.

✳ ✳ ✳

This is Creator speaking. What a marvelous journey it has been this evening! Life is an exploration. If you really look, you will see that there is so much beauty. What happened here is one simple thing. Right now, you are focused on finding light, and you are finding it.

Water has been on Earth for more than 4 billion years. Everything was here, but now you focus on the light, so more light is coming into you. When you teach, there is only one thing to teach. It is simple: You get what you focus on. When you focus on God, you get God. When you focus on something else, you get that something else. Blessings.

✳ ✳ ✳

Release Addictions

We are the angelic presence known as Beihiyud, the angel who works with addictions. Everyone has some form of addiction, whether they know it or not. The addiction could be to thoughts, behavior, or an emotional reaction or response. Many people have addictions to an attitude, such as thinking, "Life is suffering. I have to work hard to be successful or to make something out of my life." Their belief system is so addicted that they train themselves and they push themselves and others.

People can be addicted to other human beings, places, and even clothing. You can be addicted to love. Addiction is different from preferences. If you have too much attachment to something, that is addiction. All addictions come from inner emptiness.

Addictions can drive you as you seek to fulfill them through any means. Addictions can become a swirling energy shaped something like a snake. This energy always wants to consume more and more and more. The only way the snake can feed its appetite is by creating more and more addiction. Ask yourself, "What am I addicted to?" You will see there is some other need you are trying to fulfill by having this addiction. You could be addicted to your teacher, your guru, or a spiritual master. The only one you have to be addicted to is God.

Ask, "Why am I addicted, and what is the underlying theme behind the addiction? What is lacking in my life that creates this addiction?" Some people are addicted to excelling. They work very hard and are addicted to success. Some people are addicted to failure, so they create failing experiences. Some are addicted to the Internet and social media.

When you are addicted, you sabotage the energy within your brain, and your pineal gland closes. Your heart closes. The chakras inside your soul close. When you are addicted, you rarely do things in a new way. You repeat things. This gives you a kick. Some people are driven by an addiction to suffering and sorrow. Some people say life is boring because they are addicted to drama.

You can carry addictions from other lifetimes and your family lineage. These can be thought patterns that a family holds as truth. For example, many Christian families say, "Jesus is the savior who died for our sins." Some people are addicted to obedience. You must have obedience, but it must be balanced with individuality, not an exercise in giving your power away. Most addiction to authority comes from past lives, especially those in which you were forced to be obedient to a ruler, a higher authority, a tax collector, or a landlord. You must ask that all these energies be removed from your etheric level.

Some people are born again and again into a specific group. Military people are repeatedly born as warriors and are addicted to war. People who become police are born again and again as police so that they can control others. This is also an addiction.

Unless you remove your addictions, ascension cannot take place. We encourage you to discover your addictions and determine how many you brought from past lives. Ask that all addiction energy within your chakras, pineal gland, heart, and soul be removed. You will see a shift right away, and you will feel vibrations in your toes and fingers.

You also carry sexual addiction energy. This is the addiction to having sex with multiple partners in the hope that you can find yourself. This is impossible. Sex should be enjoyed, for it is the best fun you can have with your body, but it is a sacred union. It is not an animalistic instinct you use to manipulate others. Many people carry addictions in their sexual organs. Ask whether you have this energy within you, and if you do, ask that it be removed.

Another addictive energy is the attachment to a parent. You love your parents, but attachment, such as constantly seeking your mother's love without being yourself, is very different.

Love your children as much as you can, especially when they are young, but allow them to grow up. If you watch every move your children make and try to control them, you are too attached to them. You might think you do this from love, but love comes with wisdom and discretion.

Do not be addicted to anything. Enjoy everything, but do not become attached or addicted because the chakras and the pineal gland are then blocked. One easy way to remove addiction energy is through dance movements. If you are consciously aware of attachments, dance the energy away. You will feel energy move out through your feet and into the ground.

You can also sit or stand in water up to your waist. Cup water in your hands, and say, "I release all the energies from the attachments that are still in my pineal gland into this water so that it will be transmuted." Pour that water over your head.

As you grow to higher levels of mastery, you will need to clear more and more from deeper and deeper parts of you. A shamanic practice for expelling addiction is to burn it. You say, "I release all addictions still affecting me, whether I am aware of them or not. I release them into the fire." Visualize a fire coming into you and burning the energy away.

Many addictions are attached to your spinal column. The spinal column is one of the most important parts of the body. Karmic energy, attachments, and addictions all exist here. You can even have addictions to fear and bad luck. You must ask whether this is an original creation or an addiction.

✳ ✳ ✳

Are there any addictions that serve us? Are there any positive addictions or are all addictions bad?

This is Archangel Michael. There are positive addictions you can cultivate and make your reality, such as addiction to joyful creation, grace, appreciation, finding only the good in others, loving service, kindness, all good things in life, the cocreative process, and cocreating only benevolent experiences.

When we get rid of an addiction, should we ask that only the addictions that are not serving us go?

Exactly. Then you can ask that the positive addictions you want to retain be strengthened.

How do we become more aware of our addictions?

Look at your experiences, what you create, and why you do certain things. How do you respond or react? What makes you react in every situation and condition in your life? In this self-observation, you will see your addictions. Does your attachment come from the past, or is it an addiction you have cultivated in this lifetime for survival? Most addictions come from a place of survival. "If I do not do 'this,' it will be taken away from me. I have to hold on to it at any cost."

Because we have so many addictions, should we call these angels once a day or a few times a week?

You will know when to do it, and you will see a shift. You will start to do things in a new way. You will start to think differently. The paradigm will shift for you. It will be an inward shift, a cellular shift, and you will know you are releasing an attachment or an addiction.

Some people are very addicted to coffee, and others are addicted to tea. Some people are addicted to ceremonies, and some are addicted to workshops. (They are called workshop junkies.) Where does this need come from? Something drives them to seek instruction. If you can fulfill a need, perhaps your addiction will shift. Ninety-nine percent of addiction is a need that comes from an empty part of you.

The people of Israel have an addiction to the land and to the idea that Jerusalem belongs to the chosen ones. They have killed other people. During Israeli weddings, they break a glass so that they will not forget Jerusalem. It is their culture. Look at such situations, and say, "I release all cultural addictions that I have brought forth or that have been instilled in me."

* * *

Release Fear of God

Blessings, my dear family. I am Esausraham. The human race understands very little about God, and that understanding is incorrect or inappropriate. There are glimpses of understanding, but about 90 percent of human understanding of God comes from old belief systems. The Creator has said, "You are God incarnate." This is a true statement, for God is much bigger than you can conceive. God cannot be described. God is a process. God is not a specific being or thing. God is an energy that is continuously in motion and creates everything you see. God can never be described.

Most of you have imprints about what God should be. You have been taught that God is either a female or a male in the likeness of human beings. This has been instilled in you, and you do the same to your children. This can be a warmongering God, an angry God who punishes you when you do not do the right thing. If you do not sing the right chants, you cannot attain liberation. If you do not perform the right ceremonies, you cannot go to heaven.

All religions have flaws and weaknesses. What you have been told goes deep into your subconscious and becomes your reality. That reality plays out when you go to temple, shrine, church, mosque, or synagogue. You see and experience God the way you have been taught in accord with what is in your subconscious mind. You never experience the truth, the process of God, because you have been programmed with an energy pattern and belief system from your parents, religious teachers, and storybooks. This energy pattern and false belief system are stored behind the third eye, and from there, they are distributed to both ears, the mouth, the throat, and the base chakra, where it gets stuck. Your experience of God becomes very limited. There is a simple way to release the energy and false belief systems, but how long it will take depends on how many lifetimes you have carried them and how strong the imprints are.

Close your eyes, and visualize a small trickle of clear water pouring into your third eye. You are lying down, and someone is gently pouring crystal clear water into your third eye. It flows through your ears, into your mouth, and down your throat. You feel no discomfort because this energy is poured very gently. Make the intention that all false belief systems you hold are flushed out of you and from all your realities, especially the cellular imprints in your mental, emotional, and spiritual bodies.

You feel energy in your hands as these imprints leave your body. The unawakened chakras start to open. The healing chakras in your fingernails activate, and you feel energy there. Allow this. As the beautiful water pours into your third eye, some drips onto your forehead. This is also to remove false belief systems. You feel refreshed and have a remembrance of all that is the Creator. A sacredness comes into you that is absolute clarity, a clear mind without fear.

Archangels Metatron, Michael, Raphael, and Gabriel have an ashram on the inner planes. They have made a beautiful temple called the Temple of the Angelic Heart.

Go to the Temple of the Angelic Heart. There is a cubicle. Sit inside the cubicle, and see energy move clockwise around you. This creates cleansing and purifying waves of energy in your heart. Many negative energies you carry about God, such as anger or disappointment, will be pushed out.

See circling energy go into your heart. This circle becomes a spiral and grows larger and larger. Say, "I ask for the opening of the angelic heart within me. I hold the pure vibrations of the angelic heart, and I anchor them in my heart as a permanent reality from this moment and forevermore."

Go to the Temple of the Angelic Heart daily, especially when you are anxious or want to release sadness, sorrow, or similar emotions. This will greatly support you in opening your heart. Breathe it in.

If you do this clearing for the next four weeks, your energy will increase. You will be able to partake of its coming into your reality in a much more profound way because you will have released many fear-based imprints about God. When this is released, a void is created, and a new energy will fill it. You will feel grand indeed.

❋　　❋　　❋

Many artists have depicted God as a white father figure. Our culture's belief is mostly based on the Bible, which tells us of a wrathful God. How do we deal with that when we're trying to find our own image?

I am Archangel Michael. An artist depicts God in his or her own way, and that interpretation can become a cultural truth. In India, there are statues that represent God. If you are a devotee and your family worships this way, that affects you, and you think of God in that likeness. Misunderstandings of God are imprinted through cultural and religious belief systems. Many people believe angels have wings. Angels do not have wings. People try to depict the purity of an angel, and this is the only way they know how to show an angelic presence.

I still wonder what we are supposed to think about the Bible, which we are told is infallible truth. I have always had a hard time with that, especially the Old Testament.

Most of the teachings in the Bible were written long after Jesus passed away. They were passed from one hand to another almost seventy years later. There are some beautiful, inspiring messages in the Bible. Take what is best, and release the rest. If you want to read the Bible, read the Gospel of Thomas. You will feel the energy.

We ask you to work with this because your understanding must move beyond any religious belief systems imprinted into you. You can have a direct experience of the Divine within you. If you retain a belief system that God should be a particular way, you will be disappointed. If you are open, you will have wonderful experiences.

This is one of the biggest shifts people have when they ascend or pass away. They realize right away what Creator or God energy is. When this happens, their perceptions shift immensely. This is what happens with ascension: Your perceptions become larger than life. Blessings, blessings, and blessings.

CHAPTER EIGHT

Spiritual Cosmology

Angel Sribonato, Archangel Michael, and Archangel Metatron

Hello, my name is Sribonato. Archangel Michael asked me to speak. I am here to give you an understanding of who I am and my role. I hold all the spiritual principles of this universe. Many spiritual lineages of this universe branch from me. On the Earth plane, spiritual principles began with the Melchizedek school, and from it, the House of David emerged. I hold spiritual principles for the entire universe. Where will you find me? Everywhere, for I am one of the Council of Twelve. Good day to all of you.

Could you explain the House of David and its importance?

The House of David is an ancient lineage that came from the Melchizedek Order. It brought forth an understanding of spiritual evolution on this planet. All religions originated from the Melchizedek Order. Melchizedek is the master of this universe who is entrusted with the development of it, which Earth is only a small part of. The House of David was created to bring understanding to the Earth plane, but it also exists on other planets and in other realities.

In the Pleiades, Master Jesus is from the House of David, but his Pleiadian name is Sananda. The House of David played a major part in bringing forth higher consciousness to the planet. When you look closely at the House of David and its emblems, you can see that they are similar to the ancient Indian traditions of Hinduism. The Star of David is a combination of many stars, stars within stars within stars.

Are Hebrew letters found in other star systems?

Hebrew is a galactic language from another reality.

※ ※ ※

The Book of Records and the Twelve Universes

Hello, blessed ones. This is Archangel Michael. We encourage you to communicate with us in this window of opportunity. We are overjoyed when this happens because we miss you as much as you miss us. It is always a two-way street. Now I will leave the door open for any communication from my brothers and sisters. I encourage you to be open for discussion and questions.

Is the Book of Records the same as the akashic records?

It is not the akashic record. It is much bigger. The akashic record is just one part of the Book of Records. You can also call it the Universal Book of Records. The akashic record is only one part of history of akash in this dimension in this galaxy or star system. We live not only in this galaxy but in other universes as well. The Book of Records contains information from other universes.

Does the Book of Records record all our previous and future incarnations wherever we are in the universe?

Yes. You must remember, there are many universes and many creators of other universes.

When we address the Creator, we really address the Creator of the universe and dimension we live in. Is that correct?

Yes, this universe. But we suggest you expand to connect with the twelve universes.

Would you explain that?

It is worthwhile to study and examine the twelve universes that support this one. There is a council of creators that supports the evolution of this universe and this Creator. This is why it has been said, "You are, and I shall be that I shall be forever." If this universe disappeared, you would still exist because you are part of the entire spectrum of twelve universes. It is time to open to higher perceptual realities. There is much more. Now Metatron is here.

＊　　＊　　＊

Hello, dear ones. I know we are challenging your minds, just as teachers challenge your minds to pull out knowledge from inside. This is what we are trying to do. We do not give you all the information. There is so much more.

We ask you to look at these things. When you begin to communicate with the council of creators, you will see how each member can be part of several councils, similar to the board members of a corporation. The president of one company can be a board member of other companies. This Creator is a board member in other creations, and other creators are board members in this creation. Each brings the highest understanding to support the whole. Other creators support your Creator, and your Creator supports other creators.

＊　　＊　　＊

Is there a Supreme Creator who is in charge of the whole works?
I am Archangel Michael. Yes there is a Supreme Creator, the big boss of everything. That is for another time.

＊　　＊　　＊

The Power of Fridays

This is Archangel Metatron. Do you know that Friday is a sacred day? It is sacred in Israel, India, Islamic countries, and places where Tibetan Buddhism is practiced because it has a special energy. Each day has a specific vibrational frequency, and Friday's is the energy of completion and new beginnings.

The energies of death and rebirth happen on Fridays. In many cultures, people fast on Friday. This is the energy of the goddess. When you want to create something new in your life, think about beginning it on a Friday, when you can find the energy with the highest potential to create your new reality. Blessings.

CHAPTER NINE

Ascension Practices

Angel Rahmel, Archangel Michael, Angel Maharom, Angel Manna,
Angel Zagzagel, Angel Ragoan, Lord Melchizedek, Archangel Metatron,
Angel Sahuecae, Archangel Gabriel, and Angel Seetreme

My name is Rahmel. I am the angel of bandwidth. Everything in life has
bandwidth. Bandwidth makes your life linear. Without it, there would be
no beginning and no end. One sentence would flow into another without
a gap. Bandwidth defines how you function as a society and as human
beings, and it is artificially created because of the nature of karma.

People believe they need bandwidth to bring balance to the universe.
They believe that without it, there would be no gaps, and you would feel
as if your life were in turmoil and upside down. This is false. Without
bandwidth, your life would become cyclical. This is similar to a circular building that deflects the forces of nature in a hurricane or tsunami.
When there is no bandwidth, your life cycles like a beautiful fountain,
and nothing affects it.

Reduce Bandwidth

There are two tiny balls of energy inside your temples. (In some cultures,
people paint their temples. In Ethiopia, they tattoo them.) This is a very
delicate location of psychic ability. *Bring your attention to these two balls of
light in your temples. Imagine that they are spinning, and a beam of light connects one to the other, creating a bridge of light. The front of your head slowly
draws back to your ascension chakra and into the portal of your back. Allow
this energy to flow.*

Within seven days of activating this energy in your temples by working with it in your meditation, you will see a dramatic reduction in the

linear world's power to affect you. You will see a continuum in everything you do, who you are, and most importantly, what you experience. The concept of "I" slowly shifts because there will be no gap, and the concept of "we" becomes more prominent. You will experience all creation without a gap. You are one.

✳ ✳ ✳

Hello, this is Archangel Michael. Did you enjoy Rahmel? Please feel free to ask questions.

Rahmel said that he is the angel of bandwidth, but actually he is he the angel to prevent bandwidth, so we can have no gap. Is that correct?

This angel can support you to remove the gap so that you can experience everything as a part of continuous creation and stop doing one thing and then moving on to something else. This is how to remove bandwidth. Although you still have a gap in a larger sense, you will see that there is no separation.

Bandwidth is separation. This is how the world was designed to bring forth your karmic lessons. You can only experience karmic lessons through bandwidth, but you no longer need this. When you remove the separation, your karma loses its power, and there is no karma to work on. Some cultures still need it because they have to go through certain experiences.

Do you know why you have karma? At the deepest level, there is only one reason. It is not because of the law of cause and effect, which is what everyone thinks. Karma was created so that you can learn compassion. God is compassion. You learn compassion by breaking your heart over and over. When you learn compassion without karma, you experience me.

The United States used to have compassion for others. It stood on principle. There was talk about liberty and freedom, but the United States also had compassion for people who suffered. When tragic events happened in the world, America would rush to help. Many things, such as the Red Cross and other charities, started there. America gave and gave, and because of that, it was the greatest and most prosperous country. But it has changed. It was one of the most envied countries in the world, and it stood by others in times of need. This may not be true now, but it once was. Compassion creates greatness in human beings and in nations.

✳ ✳ ✳

Higher Dimensional Realities

My name is Maharom, and I am the angel of dreams. You live in other realities when you dream, and you frequently travel to places of healing, learning, interacting, and resting. You often have vivid dreams, but when you wake, the energy is gone and you no longer remember what happened. This is as it should be. If you were to remember all your dreams, it would confuse you because realities merge in your dreams. This would be too much for a linear, logical mind. You were designed to not remember your dreams. Otherwise it would be overwhelming.

You also dream celestial dreams, and you work, live, and create karma through interactions in other realities because the laws of cause and effect operate throughout the universe. When you connect with celestial dreams, you take the highest good from that reality and bring it into your reality on Earth. You can also program your dreams so that what you seek is given to you from other realities and brought into this reality. When you seek a solution to a problem, it has already been solved in another reality long ago. You can bring that solution into your present reality by asking for it.

There are sensors, or portals, underneath your eyes near the bridge of the nose. Your eyebrows are also sensors. Some people shave their eyebrows, but we suggest not doing this because they sense what you need to see and are nerve receptors for the brain that give commands to the eyes to see what is there.

Before you go to sleep, communicate with your eyebrows. Say, "I ask to be connected with celestial dreams in my other realities all the way to the tenth and eleventh dimensions." In those dimensions, your dreaming and living states become one. You are in a very high frequency, creating in a very high reality that has only benevolent creations. Your present-day life is affected by what you do up to the seventh dimension, but from there to the eleventh dimension, you are in a celestial dream. There is no separation. You are one. Your understanding of yourself and the universe is at a very high level.

Call for these realities to transfer into your personal dream state through your eyebrows. When you wake up in the morning, you will sense that you dreamed or traveled to other realities. You might not fully remember these experiences, but the pieces will slowly come together for you. New ideas and inspirations will arise. You will attract new friendships with your soul family and like-minded people. These dreams are especially good for problem solving.

You can also use your dreams to connect with your guides. Everyone dreams. You can connect with the dreams of Archangel Gabriel, Master Jesus, or Master Kuthumi. Can you envision where this can lead you? You do this by asking and connecting through your eyebrows. Since the masters are in a higher reality, their dreams are of higher reality and higher frequency. You can connect with the energy of a master by interlinking your chakras and your dreams with those of the master. Most masters dream of unity consciousness and oneness. Your life will never be the same. Blessings, this is Angel Maharom.

❋　　❋　　❋

This is Archangel Michael. Dear family, what this angel brought is very profound. Connecting with the dreams of masters can shift your life immeasurably. It will take your soul into the heavens, for the dreams of masters bring peace to this land and create new universes and frequencies. You will fly with the masters. What a gift! Remember, in the dream state, you are not in third-dimensional reality; you are in a parallel universe.

Do we have the same connections to our ascended masters and celestial guides?

Yes, in a much more profound way. You are one with them.

It seems to me that you could have direct experience of a master's consciousness.

Of course! This is where we want you to come to an understanding that you can have a direct experience of a master's consciousness. The world is moving toward understanding this.

This is what we've wanted all our lives! It is a profound inner awakening of our individual souls.

You are ready. That is why you have been brought forth.

When you talk about a master's consciousness, do you mean we can choose the master we want to connect with?

Of course! Choose a master who is appropriate for you and who is one of your guides. We are happy that you are enjoying today's session because we are taking this teaching to a very high level of consciousness and giving you tools to work with.

Remember that everyone is dreaming all the time. Through dreams, you create your reality. Everything takes a break to sleep and rejuvenate — every human being, every ascended master, everything. This is a push and pull that stops and goes. The stopping time is the dream state. In the dream state, you rejuvenate and fine-tune your blueprint. When you connect in a dream state, you connect at a very high level, and it is fun. We encourage you to work in different dream states with different beings. Blessings.

※　※　※

Support Ascension with Food Choices

Blessings. We are the angels of food, Manna. In the Hebrew and Christian traditions, "manna" simply means food. When the Israelites walked out of Egypt and to the Holy Land, they were fed manna, or food that came from the sky.

Today we wish to talk about food and its role in your evolution. You have heard the expression, "You are what you eat." There is much more to that concept. The vibrations of food affect your body, your mind, and your consciousness.

You can incorporate different types of food into a balanced and healthy diet. Foods that have leaves, like sage or spinach, can be very beneficial. There are many different types of spinach, and you may want to try baby spinach. One kind has a soft purple or burgundy color. It is a food of the gods. It can regenerate many different organs in your body and cleanse your blood stream and your mental body.

The foods children require differ from those adults require. Similarly, when you move higher and higher in your reality or into your higher self, you must adjust your food to reflect this new reality. Ask what kind of food can support you at this time in your spiritual growth. You must choose what is best for you depending on your body type and the condition you are in.

Generally, leaves support you because they take in the energy of the

Great Central Sun and are connected by roots to the ground. They are a very balanced, wholesome food. Angels touch and bless leaves. They have the capacity to transform emotions by sending energy to your tongue. Energy can be sent from your tongue to cleanse your emotional body. There are chakras beneath the tongue. Leaves transform emotional energy more than other vegetables. Experiment to see which leaves support you.

Leaves can also support digestion and elimination and are very helpful with arthritis, eye problems, and foot fungus. Leaves can do much. You can wrap food in a leaf, leave it in the sun for some time, and then eat it. The food will take on the qualities of the leaf. We encourage you to try this. People in many parts of the world wrap their food in leaves and place it underground. The balance of Earth and heaven energies provides vitality. You may also want to eat quail eggs.

We would like to give you a few ideas about foods that can help you maintain your vibrational frequency. You can try cantaloupe, papaya (one or two slices in the early morning), small burgundy-colored grapes, small cherries (orange-red, not purple), sheep's milk, sweet potato, tapioca (a small portion), sea cucumber, bamboo shoots, and lotus root. These should be sautéed and not fried. Small figs and dates are good. You can steam baby spinach with grated carrots. This will support your stomach, liver, heart, and the lining of your intestines. It can also help with your sense of smell. Try a small piece of garlic, either raw or roasted. Have lime juice in the morning in hot water with a drop or two of honey. This is very good for losing weight, giving you energy, or detoxifying. Try cabbage juice, small baby broccoli, baby corn (as fresh as possible), and beetroot (one or two pieces daily). These foods can support maintaining your vibrational frequency and the clarity of your mind.

Ascension is a shift in consciousness within your mind. It is an expansion of your mind, an explosion of light there that creates and opens a new reality within you. A time lock in your mind opens. Work with these foods to determine whether they support you. You will experience a shift in your energy and vibration, a sense of lightness, and most importantly, a sense of detachment.

Many of the normal foods you eat will become less palatable. You will eat less and less. Your taste buds change because your emotional body changes. Some foods have more emotional energy than others, meaning they have more feminine qualities and energy. The feminine is usually associated with emotions and the forces of creation. Most of this food is feminine.

You will begin to detach. To ascend, you must be detached from everything in third-dimensional reality. You have prepared for the explosion in your mind, the shift in your reality. These foods can help you come to this place. We are the energy of the angels of food, called Manna.

❋ ❋ ❋

This is Archangel Michael. Now we encourage you to ask questions.

This is a very timely message for me because I have type 2 diabetes and nothing I eat is appealing anymore.

Your body has shifted. All the food you used to enjoy does not appeal to you anymore because of the shift in your emotional body. Eating raw food will help you clear your emotions. You will release much karmic energy not only from this lifetime but from others as well.

❋ ❋ ❋

Experience the Flame of the Burning Bush

Hello, my family, this is Angel Zagzagel. I am the angel of the burning bush. There have been many interpretations of the burning bush that appeared to Moses. Some said it was an angel. We are a collective angelic consciousness who appeared to Moses. You can call the burning bush and have your own experience with it. We encourage you to do this. You are all like Moses. He came to liberate his people. How did Moses do that? First he liberated his own mind. I am going to call all of you the Moseses of the present generation who are leading people not out of Egypt but out of the darkness of the Earth plane. You are all called to do that; otherwise, you would not be here. We offer you the gift of the burning bush. You can call on the burning bush in your meditation.

Make sure that you are in a very relaxed, comfortable, and powerful place, for this is a powerful experience. Close your eyes, and rest both forearms gently on your solar plexus. Gently breathe from this area. Keep breathing. You might feel some warmth coming into your arms or your solar plexus or another sensation. Allow it.

[Chants: Ahhhh, ahhhh, ahhhh.] Now I, the angel of the burning bush, step in front of you and put my hands on top of yours, emitting a brilliant orange light into your hands and solar plexus. See an orange flame shoot up from your solar plexus area becoming bigger and bigger and bigger. Allow it to become bigger than you. Ask three questions of this flame, questions you might already have asked for eons and continue to ask: "Who am I? Where am I from? What is my purpose?"

The burning bush will answer your questions. When you ask, "Who am I?" see the flame engrave the answer on a tablet designed for you. When you ask, "Where am I from?" again see the flame engrave the answer on a tablet. When you ask, "What is my life purpose?" once more, see the answer engraved in the stone.

Allow this transformation to take place. I am the flame. I am the answer. I am the question. I am All That Is. I am the messenger of the mighty high Elohim. [Chants: Elohiiiim, Elohiiiim, Elohiiiim.] Be in this space — in the stillness of this space, in the sacredness of this space, and in the warmth of this space. I will withdraw my energy slowly. We ask that you stay in this space for a moment more. We are the angels of the burning bush. We bless every one of you.

When you work with this flame daily, you will find the answer you seek. We are the messengers of the Elohim, and we bring understanding to human beings who sincerely ask. Blessings, blessings, blessings.

✳   ✳   ✳

Dear ones, what you experienced is the same energy that Moses experienced, but Moses's experience was amplified many thousands of times because he had a larger role to play. This energy can transform you just as it transformed Brother Moses, for all of you are the vanguards of a transformational shift to lead people out of darkness. Brother Moses is one of the most important players during this transitioning process. Call on this brother. Work with the sacred flame of the Elohim and his angels. You will experience a great shift.

You know, the fifth dimension is not something far away. It is in your mind. It is not somewhere outside of you. It is a part of your brain. When you work with this energy, this flame, the veil becomes thinner and thinner and completely burns out. Then you are automatically in the fifth dimension. When you work with this flame daily, you will also see that the energy you spent and the energy you gathered will last for long periods in your earthly life, and you will also experience healing on a cellular level and the end of aging. This flame has the capacity to stop aging, to stop the reproduction of cells that create health problems in your body. The priorities in your life will become clearer, and what you must look for and work for will become apparent.

This flame is from a larger flame from another reality. The violet flame of transformation of Saint Germain is part of this flame. This flame came from another reality, from another planet in the Pleiades. Blessings, this is Archangel Michael.

✳   ✳   ✳

Remove Your Energetic Thorns

Hello. My name is Ragoan. I am the angel of the rose. Greetings and love to you. May you all awaken the rose within you. Human beings behave and act like roses. Although you carry much beauty, you also have thorns. You allow others to enjoy your beauty from afar, but if they come too close, you can prick them.

Perhaps you have heard of experiments in which people talked to rosebushes. The plants felt comfortable and did not develop thorns. Why do humans have thorns? You might say for self-protection. Self-protection is based on a false belief system rooted in fear and survival. You do not need thorns. The belief that people compete with each other is based on the illusion of superiority. By maintaining your thorns, you create a false belief system about your specialness. Make a concentrated effort to remove your thorns so that all who come into your energy field can enjoy your beauty. Ask where your thoughts come from: a place of pure inner beauty that is the sacred divine within you or a place of thorns and self-survival.

It has been said that people do not love each other. Mothers and fathers do not love their children. They love themselves through their children. Ask whether the expression of love you exhibit is self-love or true love. When you remove the walls you have created, you will express love for what love is, not as love for yourselves through other people. Roses are here to learn this life lesson along with human beings. We angels help the roses heal this issue too.

You can call on us to heal issues, and the healing will remove the energetic thorns within you. These thorns are embedded in your intestinal area. Focus your attention there.

Close your eyes, and see a beautiful turquoise light in your intestinal area. See light shoot from there and flow down through your feet into the ground. Allow this turquoise light to flow through the intestinal area and downward. Feel a sense of self-sufficiency: "I can stand on my own." You value and love yourself. Walls come down. You allow other people to get close to you. You do not seek to love yourself through other people, and you do not engage other people with an ulterior motive. You come from a place in the fullness of you, and the fragrance of the flower within you will touch many. They will honor you for it. Call on us, and we will work with you.

Use Rose Energy to Attract Love, Friendship, and Peace

You can use roses to attract a partner or a friend. Take one pink rose petal and one red rose petal. Put them in a glass of crystal clear water, and let it steep for some time. Then drink the water and swallow the petals. The petals will not damage your physical body. You will absorb the vibration of the rose petals, and you will feel better about yourself. You can also drop a rose petal into the food you cook. Many cultures have used rose petals in cooking. Or you can put rose petals underneath your pillow to feel the vibrations of love when you go to sleep. See whether this supports you.

You can take three red rose petals and place them on the top of your head, placing some space between each, and then meditate. You will feel vibrations coming into your head. You will begin to feel good about yourself and have a sense of upliftment.

The universal rose energy is very beautiful. It is pink. You can call forth the universal rose energy. In your meditation, ask for the activation of the universal rose. This activation is done by the goddesses who hold the frequency of the feminine. If you are really keen to work more, you can call on sister Mary Magdalene, and she can initiate you into the order of the roses. She is supported by Mother Mary, Isis, and Gaia.

When you work with the universal rose energy, you work with the frequency of Lord Melchizedek. The Star of David is embedded within the universal rose. The flower of life comes from the universal rose. This is given only when you are ready and you request this in your meditation.

We encourage you to work with rose petals. You will see magic in your lives. Blessings.

※　　　※　　　※

Blessings. This is Lord Melchizedek. Archangel Michael and Angel Ragoan requested that I speak about the universal rose. The universal rose represents universal love, wisdom, and beauty. My twelve disciples are called the twelve Melchizedek disciples. They distribute the energy of the universal rose into this and other planets every day. What happens on Earth has a significant implication for the entire universe. You have been told this before. This is why so many watch and wait to see what will happen on the Earth plane, for what is really happening is the making of a road map for the 1,000 years of peace that are coming to the planet, the golden consciousness. This starts with the activation of the universal rose energy within your heart. You will identify yourself as a citizen of not only a state or county but the universe.

Activate the Universal Rose

Close your eyes, and bring your attention to your heart. See a large, beautiful pink rose there. My disciples and I are beaming energy into this rose. See this rose slowly open and expand. It is very large for a rose. The petals are as big as cabbage leaves. Let it expand in your heart area.

The middle of this rose contains two golden seeds. See these two seeds beam golden light that goes into and through your eyes to the other senses of your body so that you open your universal vision. The energy flows into your brain but is mainly anchored in your eyes so that you can see yourself as a universal being. Your perception of reality changes, and the structural formations your eyes are used to seeing shift. Your eyes see through geometrical patterns and interpret them in a nanosecond into the language you know and use. Everything in the universe is geometric.

When the universal rose energy is anchored into your eyes, you can see perfect sacred geometry, not a version distorted by the misuse of energy. You can see the original blueprints of how every experience should be in every situation. Because of free will, no one can say how it will appear. Nevertheless, there is an original blueprint underneath for the highest and best experience. You will see that blueprint. Let this energy fill your head and move slowly into the back of your body.

Inside the beautiful universal rose is a very small being of light. See this being of light slowly rise from the universal rose and enter your third eye. [Chants: Holy, holy, holy, holy, holy, holy.] See this being merge with you. You are one. Feel its presence. Breathe. You feel the energy flow through you, becoming a part of your energetic body — your physical, mental, emotional, and spiritual bodies. Anchor it underneath your feet and into the bosom of Mother Earth.

Now I, Lord Melchizedek, place a crown of roses on your head, holding the frequency of the universal rose in your energetic field, and I anchor it there permanently. [Chants: Uwa hoo, uwa hoo, uwa hoo.] Allow the energy to sink into your head and flow slowly into your neck, through your body, and into the ground. Breathe deeply three times. Gently open your eyes.

Blessings and my love to all of you, for this is a gift you have earned. You have longed for this and waited for it. You have opened this gift within you. This day is a grand day, and it will be recorded in your akash. Earth citizens, hold this light with pride, passion, and love in your hearts, for from now on, you are ambassadors. We call you light ambassadors.

✳   ✳   ✳

Hello, family. This is Archangel Michael with Angel Ragoan. We encourage you to meditate every day to activate the universal rose. You will see incredible light within your being and in the being who entered from the universal rose. This is your own I Am presence. This is you — all of you — merging with the universal you.

✳   ✳   ✳

Personal Initiations

Hello, precious ones. This is Archangel Metatron. Greetings and deep love to all of you. What you are going through in these sessions is your personal ascension initiations. In ancient times, initiations took place in temples and power spots. In the new reality, initiations take place in everyday life while you are fully involved in the world and maintain a higher vibration. Your initiation is a gift. We are overjoyed that we can share this with you. We do not share much with others because on many levels, there is no environment for us to come through. We want to say thank you.

Archangel Metatron has many names, but I have a favorite bird, the golden eagle. I am a part of the ancient Hindu God Vishnu. His mode of transportation is a flying Garuda, a big eagle. I encourage you to work with this beautiful being, for there is much it can bring forth in understanding earthly life and other dimensional realities.

There is a flower that is also very dear to me, and that is a reddish orange lotus. We encourage you to spend time focusing on the eagle in your meditation. See an eagle on the right and a beautiful lotus on the left. Both will speak to you. They are the yin and yang energy within you. They are the God/Goddess energy within you, the perfect balance between male and female. How would you like to have these two companions in your life every day, every moment? They are with you. Tap into them. Make them part of your reality.

❋   ❋   ❋

Activate the Spinal Cord Lotus

This is Archangel Michael. We have a really wonderful angel, the angel of the spinal cord, the spinal column. You have heard about the importance of the spinal column. It was described in ancient India as the stem of the lotus. When we start from the stem, the lotus blooms beautifully. This angel works to strengthen the spinal column. This angel is Sahuecae.

❋   ❋   ❋

Hello, dear family. This is Angel Sahuecae. Blessings, blessings, and blessings. I come from the planes of Lord Melchizedek, the wise and ancient one who initiated the understanding of spirit in the Earth plane.

The spinal column is an important part of the human body not only because it helps you live but also because it carries many vital functions and energy configurations from past lifetimes and life streams on other planets and in other galaxies. Your spinal column is directly connected to the mountains, the water, the trees, the dragons, and the fish, for these carry supporting energies for you. When the spinal column is blocked, you cannot remember much and you can have denseness in your energetic bodies. When your spinal column is open, cleansed, fresh, and pure, you are much more lighthearted, fun, and loving, and your understanding and perception levels are much higher.

Close your eyes, and gently bring your attention to the back of your body and your spinal column. Ask, "How open is my spinal column?" and listen for an answer. You will immediately be shown a number. Do not judge that number. It does not matter, for it can be shifted. Then ask, "How can I open it further?" You will have an intuitive sense of the answer right away.

There are fluids in your body that are directly related to your past karmic energies and past life streams, but they can be shifted. These fluids have vibrational patterns and frequencies. Say, "I give intention to shift the frequency of the fluid within me so that I can flush out past karmic energies that have completed their timeline in my life." See this fluid in your mind's eye, and release it. You may feel a vibration, an energy, a color, or a light, but do not worry.

Now say, "I bring into my spinal column fluids of the new consciousness coming from the heart of God, and I now anchor these fluids into my spinal column." See energy coming to you. Say, "I raise this new fluid within my spinal column to the top of my head." Visualize this energy going to the spinal column, into the back of the neck, and to the top of your head.

Now state, "I open the God flower within me." See a very beautiful, incredibly soft lotus open. The stem of this lotus runs through your spinal column to Mother Earth's body and anchors there. Repeat this statement three times: "I am the flower. I am its fragrance. I am beauty and love. I am." Breathe in the energy of God three times.

Dear ones, what you have brought forth from the past two sessions are new activations to raise your frequency immediately. Blessings. I am the angel of the spinal cord.

❋　　❋　　❋

Hello, blessed family. This is Archangel Gabriel. We encourage you to be gentle with yourself, for there have been great energies downloaded into you. A great activation is taking place in your spinal column and mind, so just be gentle with yourself. Simply say when you wake up in the morning, "I give intention to be nice to me today in every way. I promise to be nice to myself today in every way."

❋　　❋　　❋

Work with the Ascension Angels

This is Archangel Michael. We would like to introduce some angels who can support your ascension process. We — all guides, teachers, and ascended masters — are here to support people's ascension, but there are specialized angels and archangels who work in a certain frequency to specifically support the ascension process. It is like being in a PhD program. After you finish your coursework, you work with a professor to write your dissertation. You have all come to this level, and now there are angels and archangels to support your ascension path. You have to make the effort, do the research, find out more, and bring a new understanding so that you are awarded your PhD degree.

These angels are here to support you. We give you these names for a short initiation. One of the angels you might want to work with is named Vaarmar. Another is Eth. One is Sakgune. Another is Monaeden. Another angel is Jirhaber. The last is Madior.

Ascension Initiation

Close your eyes, and visualize six angels surrounding you. Visualize them as beautiful, pale-white energy fields. The six angels make a humming sound. They send this humming energy throughout your chakra column. [Chants: Oooo, oooo, oooo.] They place rings of light around each of your chakras. See the rings around your chakra column as white light. See a golden thread coming from your base chakra and going through the six rings all the way to your third eye and then into your head. Allow for this golden thread of light to flow.

See a bowl of water beneath your feet. See yourself step into this bowl of water. I, Archangel Michael, dip my sword of truth and wisdom into the water, turning the water into an orange light. See this light come through the soles of your feet and flow upward, shooting through your head and then falling around you. Allow for this light to flow.

The angel Vaarmar works with energy centers around your head. There are more than fifteen energy centers to activate between your neck and the top of your head. In your mind's eye, see this angel place his two hands behind your neck and activate the fifteen centers. Let any thoughts, feelings, and visualizations come through.

The Angel Eth touches your heart. Eth works with the perception of time and reality, blending all aspects of time — of the cosmos, of the changing seasons, of moon cycles, and of planetary movements. He recalibrates your heart to these sources of time.

The Angel Sakgune places his hand above your solar plexus, stimulating your stomach, bowel, and liver so that you are able to hold higher frequencies of light in these parts of your body.

Angel Monaeden places his hands between the first and the second chakras, removing the imprints of survival and poverty consciousness from the way you act, how you react, and the actions you take. He recalibrates the geometric patterns in your physical body. We will say more about that in a moment.

The Angel Jirhaber touches your knees. The chakras there represent understanding of Earth and your role and history on the Earth plane. When this happens, your understanding of the consciousness of Mother Earth becomes important, and you will be able to fully partake of the goddess wisdom she holds. This is the mother wisdom.

The last angel, Madior, touches your ankles, releasing the energy of the magnetics. You can become lighter and can hold higher frequencies of light.

There are eight sacred geometric patterns in your physical body, beginning with a sphere on top of your head (from your nose to your crown). You have other geometric patterns as well: the tetrahedron, the vesica piscis, the square, the flower of life, the octahedron, the dodeca-hedron, and the half-moon. These sacred geometric patterns resonate and regulate the energy movements in your chakra column. Your chakra column exists not only on the physical plane but also on other dimensions. Even if you work to release and activate your physical chakra column, nothing much really happens unless you balance the sacred geometry within you. The sacred geometry cuts through all barriers up to the twelfth dimension.

These angels now ask you to spread your fingers, and they place a ring on each finger and your thumbs. Eight rings represent the sacred geometric patterns in your body — circle, vesica piscis, square, tetrahedron, flower of life, octahedron, dodecahedron, and half-moon. The other two rings represent the balanced energy of heaven and Earth.

These angels now ask you to open your palms and spread your fingers. They place eight rings of light on your fingers and two on your thumbs. The rings on your fingers represent the balanced energy of the sacred geometric patterns in your physical body. The rings placed on your thumbs represent the balanced energy of heaven and Earth.

The angels also work with the great dragon Vaa, who is the king of the archetypal dragons. He holds the immense power of awakening the kundalini of Mother Earth, which is directly related to your kundalini. *See this awesome being standing in front of you and breathing his fire into your third eye. See the fire shoot up into your head, go into the ascension chakra at the back of your head, and flow through the spinal column into the ground. Ground it there. Allow this incredible being to send his light into you. Breathe. Let the energy go deep into the ground, and hold it there.*

Now the angels step back, and only the dragon Vaa is in front of you. Your chakras and your sacred geometry patterns connect energetically to the dragon's chakras, as they have similar patterns of energy. The dragon steps closer to you and touches the base of your spine with his claw, sending an incredible electric energy into your spine. Breathe it in, and allow it to flow through you. Allow it to flow through you and out of you.

The dragon steps backward. He is once again surrounded by the angels. In your mind's eye, see only light inside your body. This light is silver platinum and is shaped like an infinity sign. All your chakras have become one infinity sign. [Chants: Ahhhh, ahhhh, oooo, oooo.] Breathe three times, dear ones, and gently open your eyes.

We encourage you to call on these specialized angels, for they are your doctoral thesis specialists who can support you through the last part of the ascension process. For the next several days when you close your eyes in meditation, visualize this beautiful silver infinity sign. When you feel a drop in energy, call on the dragon Vaa. He is the head of the archetypal dragons who seeded this planet. Ask him to energize your third eye and spinal column. Be cautious, because his energy is very powerful. You must be ready to hold his incredible power. It can have a very big effect. Although you are tired, you may not be able to sleep sometimes because you have too much light in your body. Work with this energy at your own discretion. It is very powerful.

These specialist angels can take you on a large part of your journey of ascension. They can support you. Work with them for the next several days and weeks and even for years to come, and you will see an incredible amount of energy come into you. You will also understand your role as a planetary healer and your spiritual evolution. You will see beauty wherever you travel. You will carry this frequency of light and anchor it into the ground, and healing will take place.

All of you will teach ascension to others within the next three years. This is one of the paths you can take. Let us give appreciation and thanks to these wonderful angels. Make them your friends, and work with them.

Open and Activate Your Pineal Gland

Every major organ in the human body has a guardian spirit or angelic force supporting it to perform to the maximum and coordinate with other organs. Our next angel's specialty is working with the pineal gland. This angel's name is Seetreme. Let us invite the great Angel Seetreme to share his wisdom and love with you.

✳   ✳   ✳

Blessed brothers and sisters of light, we collectively hold the consciousness of the angelic being called Seetreme. We are contained as an individual, but we are a group consciousness. We thank you for the gift of sharing this truth and wisdom with you.

The pineal gland is shaped like a pinecone and is important in opening to higher consciousness. Much has been written about the pineal gland and its importance. The pineal gland was fully open in Lemurian times and during the years of golden consciousness in Atlantis. Because of misuse and misunderstanding, it has slowly shriveled, becoming very small. It now needs to be opened.

There are many ways to open the pineal gland: breathing techniques, visualizations, sacred symbols, and sound frequencies. All support the opening and flowering of the pineal gland. Because it has not been used, it has acquired a mineral cover, and as a result, the pineal gland cannot emit its true pure light. This blocks energy from reaching the brain. Brain function can deteriorate, and that can lead to Alzheimer's disease, forgetfulness, and feeling spaced-out and generally unwell in the mind. It can cause devastating effects in the bones because the spiritual energy that is the vital essence is not reaching them or the organs to keep them healthy. They lack nourishment from the pineal gland.

The pineal gland also regulates thought processes for manifestation. Energy goes from your thoughts about what you want to create and what you believe about creation to the pineal gland, which sends this message to your signature cell. From there, it is distributed to the sacred geometry patterns in your body and to your chakras and manifests in what we call reality. When the pineal gland is blocked, these manifestation processes halt.

Think about the pineal gland. When it is open, you are in the full flow of the higher frequencies called God consciousness. Every day, visualize a small light bulb in the right hemisphere of your brain glowing silver white. In your meditation, imagine this light bulb growing and beginning to emit a bluish light. The light goes from your pineal gland to your spinal column. When that happens, there will be chemical reactions in the spinal column that release cerebral fluids holding karmic patterns of energy. This energy is drained through your feet and into the ground. Much of the karmic energy that needs to be balanced is flushed out. You retain the wisdom without needing to go through the physical experiences.

Close your eyes. Bring your attention to your third eye, and visualize a blue light there. Breathe this beautiful blue light into your third eye, and exhale. As you inhale, hold your breath and visualize it going into the right hemisphere of your brain. Your brain is filled with the blue light, and energy pushes to the right hemisphere of your brain. Breathe through the third eye. Just breathe. Breathe again.

Visualize a small sacred triangle. As you breathe, the sacred triangle slowly embeds in your third eye. Send your breath through the sacred triangle into the right hemisphere of your brain. Visualize a small triangle inside the right hemisphere of your brain. On top of the triangle is a wick. A small lamp fills your entire brain with its sacred light. Continue breathing. Blue light flows into the sacred triangle, and light coming through the sacred triangle fills your brain.

When your pineal gland starts operating, it sends light into your brain, and you feel energy in your hands. The coordination of your hands is directly connected to your pineal gland. You might feel a tingling sensation or vibrations in your fingers.

Keep breathing the blue light from your third eye into the right hemisphere of your brain and into the triangle. When your pineal gland starts working and sending light, your healing ability opens considerably. Coordination of hand movements becomes much smoother and wiser. You feel as if your hand movements create benevolence. (This is the basis of mudras. Every time you use your hands, you are using the dance of hands to create specific types of energy. You are not just doing something with your hands. You are using the energy within your hands to create a specific reality. When you type, you create a

typing reality. When you drink coffee, you create that reality.) Your experi-
ences heighten. Your hands become very sensitive. Then everything you create
comes from a heightened state of awareness. You have reached and are experi-
encing the Divine within you.

Allow this energy to flow into your hands. Breathe it in. Blue light from
your third eye enters the right hemisphere into the small triangle, and a lamp
burning at the top of the right hemisphere spreads light into your brain and then
into your hands. You feel a tingling, pulsing sensation on the fingertips. Allow
this. Breathe it in. Just breathe it in. Breathe it in deeply.

Ask for Angelic Healing Light

Here is another method for activating the pineal gland. There is also
a sacred triangle above the ascension chakra on the medulla oblongata
at the back of the neck. Ask the angelic presence — especially us, Seetreme, the angels of the pineal gland — to inject liquid angelic light
into this place. This liquid angelic light will flow from the back of your
neck to the middle of your brain, activating and breathing energy into
your pineal gland, healing many imbalances, rearranging thought patterns, and removing lower frequencies of thought energy embedded in
your brain. This is only given when asked. You can request this healing
before you go to sleep, and we will work with you while you sleep. When
you wake in the morning, you will feel a different sensation.

Sometimes when the pineal gland is activated, there is a lot of energy in
the brain, and you might not be able to sleep for some time until your
body adjusts to the higher frequency. We can support you in regulating
the energies so that you can rest. The light in your pineal gland will
gather more and more momentum, and you will sleep less and less. The
density of your body will decrease, and you will need less sleep. Your body
will be fully vitalized and will hold only higher frequencies of thought
energy.

We will stand aside now. We encourage you to share your thoughts,
questions, and comments about this so that we can support you.

※　　※　　※

Does anybody have any questions? This is Archangel Michael.

Since we started this exercise, my head has been spinning. I want to shake.

Yes, dear one. You are activating the higher frequency of light. Holding a stone can support you. You might want to spend some time near a plant. If the feeling persists, place your feet in a bowl of water and say, "I drain the excess energy into this water through my feet." You will feel a difference if you stay there for five minutes. We are talking about very high frequencies when you work with this, so be gentle with yourself. If you cannot take it, say, "I'm going to stop this now. I can come back to this another time."

Can the pineal gland turn?

Of course! It turns, it spins, it grows, and it changes color.

CHAPTER TEN

Angelic Energy Practices

Angel Akatriel, Archangel Michael, and Angel Mahyon

Blessings. May the greatest love of the universe be bestowed on all of you. I am the angel of prayer and devotion. I carry the name and the energy of Akatriel.

Prayer is an important form of communication with the Creator. True prayer, said with full feeling, has the potential to be manifested in your reality. But a prayer said in fear has very little potential, for the vibration of the prayer must match its intention. Have you ever considered the vibration of your prayer when you pray? The frequency of a prayer depends on your faith and what you believe about the prayer.

Action-Based Prayer

When you truly pray, whom do you pray to? You pray to yourself. When you fold your hands in front of your heart in a prayer position, your two thumbs point toward your heart. Your palms represent the God force within you. So in truth, you pray to yourself, and since you are connected to the whole, you are a part of the whole. When you pray, the creative force automatically feels your prayer. Action-based prayer will bring the highest result.

Close your eyes, bring your hands to a prayer position in front of your heart, and breathe a beautiful turquoise color. See this turquoise color. Visualize it all over your hands. Breathe it in. Visualize a beautiful turquoise sphere on top of your head. You may pray silently about anything you like. Any prayer will do — a prayer for guidance, abundance, or anything else. Place the prayer inside the sphere above your head.

See the sphere slowly descend through your chakra column, from the soul star chakra to the crown to the third eye to the throat to the heart to the solar plexus to the sacral chakra and the base chakra. Then let this sphere of light go into your toes.

Your toes are a very important part of your body. They are not just for balancing the physical body. They have important energy points and much wisdom. They are activation points for the third DNA layer to awaken your consciousness through action. We are teaching you to pray based on action.

Feel the energy on the toes of both feet. When you feel the energy in your toes, you are inspired to take action to manifest a reality that comes from the highest parts of yourself. Use this method for one prayer at a time.

We would like you to experiment with this method of prayer for the next two weeks. We guarantee that you will see results. New ideas, inspirations, thought forms, or even actions might come to you. It is very important to have a method of prayer that is practically based for the Earth plane.

When you pray with gratitude, the Elohim pick up that prayer and create thoughts and forms so that your prayer has a great potential to manifest. When you say a prayer from a place of gratitude, the energy goes into your pineal gland. Your pineal gland is connected to the whole universe. You might sense a beam of light for a nanosecond with the beings who pick up the energy of your prayer and set to work to manifest it. They might utilize the elements, the dragons, or the energy of the Moon and Sun to manifest your prayer.

You can also use the great desert for prayer, especially if the desert is a golden earth color. Visualize a desert, and coming from a feeling of gratitude, place your prayer on the sand. See the sand blow away in all directions. This takes your intention and spreads it to the four corners of Earth — east, west, north, and south. At the appropriate time, you will feel the energy regarding your prayer rise inside of you. The desert can manifest a prayer much faster than other elements, faster than water, especially when a prayer is based on appreciation and gratitude.

Another way of praying is through giving. When you give something to someone or help somebody, such as giving food to a homeless person, you offer a prayer. This is one of the highest forms of prayer that has the capacity to transform your karma.

We encourage you to practice all forms of prayer. Take a week to practice each kind of prayer, and observe whether you have results. You will definitely see some changes.

Activate Prayer Codes

You can activate prayer codes when you bring your attention above your third eye, below the angel chakra, in the middle of your forehead. See a beautiful sun shining there. Breathe through this place, and pray there. Place your prayer in this area, and breathe out from there. This sends the energy of your prayer throughout your cells not only on the physical level but also on all levels. It has the potential to manifest your prayer very quickly.

The great master Si Baba used these methods to create and manifest a desired reality in an instant. The great teacher Paramahansa Yogananda used this method to pluck roses from the air. We encourage you to experiment with these methods and note how they benefit you and change your life.

When you do something of service, create it as a form of prayer. When you give water to plants, food to the birds, or pet your cat, this is a form of prayer. A simple thought held with feelings will shift your life very quickly. You can experience every moment as a living prayer. Jesus demonstrated this. When he walked, he was a living prayer. When he breathed, he was a living prayer. Everything he did was a living prayer.

We wish to add one more thing before we go. There is masculine prayer and feminine prayer. A masculine prayer can become a catalyst for change that needs physical energy. A feminine prayer comes from love and compassion and can also create change through compassion and kindness. Blessings, blessings, and blessings. This is Akatriel, the angel of prayer.

✳   ✳   ✳

Angelic Sound

Hello, blessed ones. This is Archangel Michael. In our sessions, we bring forth understanding for different kinds of angelic breathing, mudras, and sounds that you might find fascinating. I would like to give you a sound today. You can practice it for the next several days, and you will feel a great expansion. This sound is "kaatmaido." Repeat this daily. [Chants:

Kaatmaido. Ka–At–Maid-O.] It means "I have the peace and light of angels within me." Kaatmaido. "An angel's light is within me." You will feel energy come into and above your third eye area. [Chants: Kaatmaido. Kaatmaido.] Repeat this as many times as you want — when you walk, when you take a shower, whenever. You can repeat it loudly or softly. It does not matter. You will feel the frequency. By doing this, you are building a bridge of light between you and the angels. The angels will feed you with peace and light. We thank you once again.

✳ ✳ ✳

Find Magic and Mastery by Working with Plants

This is Mahyon. My dear brothers and sisters, it is my joy to communicate with you, for we are a group of angels working with the plant and tree kingdoms. Plants are a vital part of your evolution and of the ecosystem. People have houseplants because they are beautiful and give you support and energy, but they also have a much bigger role. Plants take on the karmic energy of human beings, and they will sacrifice their lives because they love humanity.

It is good to have a plant that you are able to connect with daily, for they have personalities and souls. You might wonder what plants are best for you. This will shift depending on your frequency, vibration, and location on your evolutionary path. For example, if you are working toward physically attaining your ascension with higher dimensional energy, then you might have a plant that differs from the kind someone would need to support healing depression.

Different people need different plants. If you live with other people, it is good to have a variety of plants, for each plant vibrates at a specific frequency to support specific people. When you go to your nursery, you must ask the plant, "Do you support me? Would you support my energy field?"

Try to find a small pine tree to grow in a pot in the house because these can be very therapeutic. They bring healing energy into an environment. The tulsi plant [holy basil] from India is considered sacred and is used in rituals and prayer ceremonies for Indian gods and goddesses. This plant supports harmony, balance, and sacredness in your environment. A willow can support healing depression and impart general well-being. The lily (called "uri" in Japan) can support awakening your inner beauty and helps you understand how each person is precious.

Plants can support raising your vibration. There are certain plants that support the transformation of energy, especially in the ascension process. This is why many cultures offer plants and flowers as gifts to the Creator.

One plant you might want to work with is lavender. Lavender can calm your emotions and open the energy within you to become a clearer channel. You understand the inspiration coming into you, and you can comprehend and utilize it. You can have lavender plants in every part of a home.

Plants take on the consciousness of the person who looks after them. When you communicate with a plant, care for it and love it. In four months, the plant will be able to answer your questions because it will have completely integrated your energy not on a personality level but on the level of your physical, mental, emotional, and spiritual bodies. Plants are very sensitive. They are fine-tuned to the sensitivity of your physical body. Make it a habit to communicate with plants every morning after you wake. Greet them, and you will feel their love and communication.

If you have writer's block, sit near a plant. Meditate with it for ten minutes, and see green light flowing into your hands and filling you. Then you will be able to write, for plants can open your creativity, especially at a time and place where there is great opportunity to exhibit your soul talent. Is your talent managing, writing, communicating, or public speaking? Is it bringing people together so that they can listen?

We encourage you to communicate with a plant every day. When in doubt, place your hand above the leaves, and you will feel vibrations. When you feel the vibrations, simply ask what you need to know, and the plant will answer you. It will take three to four months for the plant to fully integrate your energy. This requires two processes: loving the plant and caring for it. When the plant knows you care for it, it will reveal its secrets.

Plant spirits are directly connected to the solar kingdom. The solar devas create magic and mastery. You must master solar kingdom energy for true magic to happen. These are the teachings of Saint Germain and Lord Merlin. True magic takes place through understanding nature spirits and in transforming the energy of nature into what you want to create.

The first step is to get in touch with the plant spirits and work with them. You will integrate the energy of the plant's spirit, which is the beginning of magic.

Plants Strengthen Your Bond with God

There are plants you can keep anywhere you need balanced energy. If you had ten or twelve plants in a delivery room where babies are born, they would impart the energy of the sacredness of birth. A company's boardroom has energy of structure and hierarchy, and some people are not able to speak up. Plants could calm everyone and instill a sense of peace, love, and unity consciousness.

Ask your surgeon whether he or she would like to have some plants in the operating theater. If someone were having a heart operation, having three or four plants near could absorb a lot of the discomforting pain energy. The patient would have less pain and less need for medication. The patient would be much more conscious, and healing would take place more quickly.

Plants placed in a train station or an airport can create harmony. So many people are coming and going. Plants can balance these energies. A classroom with plants might have less violence. The children could be more receptive to what the teacher says because the plants would calm their minds. Plants work on the unconscious mind, bringing a sense of calm.

Although plants have green leaves, they emit a golden-green light that has a tint of purple. Breathe this light in, and you will start integrating with plants; you will start being like a plant. Every life form is a unique expression of God. Human beings could manifest their true potentials. You are united with all creation. You are individual aspects, but you are nevertheless part of the whole. When plant consciousness is integrated within you, you make it part of your reality. What a beautiful concept.

We encourage you to work with plants by sitting with them, meditating with them, communicating with them, and sending love to them to strengthen the bond between you and Creator. This will calm your mind because the energy from the plant will go into your chakras. When it goes into your base chakra, the feelings of being insecure and fear-driven will diminish.

As you meditate in front of a plant, see the golden-green light with a tinge of soft purple enter your base chakra. Let it fill with this color, and the energy will flow back to the plant like an infinity sign. It will also go into the second and third chakras. This will start to break survival consciousness. You will no longer operate from a place of survival, thinking, "Me, me, me." Instead, you will be in a place of creation with the joyful aspects of yourself because almost all plants are joyful. Even when they are put in horrible conditions, they emit serene energy.

When you wake up, you can say, "Plant, I ask you to share your serene energy with me." Breathe the plant into your lower three chakras. You might send the energy through your feet into the earth, grounding it there. Within three to six months, your spirit will appear in your mind's eye, for each plant has a deva spirit working in connection with Helios and Vesta, the solar angels. You will start vibrating on the solar level. Your solar chakras will open. Your heart chakra will vibrate with Earth's heart chakra and the solar heart chakra. Every aspect of you will be uplifted in a gentle and benevolent way. You will be integrated at a very high level.

We encourage you to work with plants every day to see the shift. You will notice a gentleness and peacefulness come into you. You will move at a slower pace. Your life will become calmer. You will be able to think clearly and get more things done in less time. You will be able to hold your equilibrium. You will not lose your calm, and you will retain your power. This is Mahyon.

✳   ✳   ✳

This is Archangel Michael. Different plants will come into your life. When you are looking for a job, there is a plant that can support you. The plant will not bring a job to you, but it can inspire you so that you will take action to manifest a job. There are plants that are good for marriage. Some people suffer marriage blues before they commit. They become frightened and nervous because they feel as if they are losing their freedom. A plant can support healing that feeling before a wedding. Talk to it about eleven days before the wedding, and the plant will absorb all your anxiety.

We encourage you to think about placing three plants in the corners of a delivery room to support the babies coming into the world. It will ease the pain of separation and allow the babies to adjust to the environment much easier. Plants help babies open their lungs to breathe easily. We encourage you to ask doctors and midwives whether they would like to have plants wherever children are born.

Mudras for Angelic Support

Archangel Michael

Mudras are energetic positions that can create specific vibrational frequencies to bring about desired changes in your life. They were practiced during the times of Lemuria, and some were used by people of the Mayan culture. These mudras were originally encoded into the secret codes of Mother Earth. They can liberate your mind very quickly. The time has now come for them to be released because humanity is ready for them.

Find the Joy of Living in the Present Moment

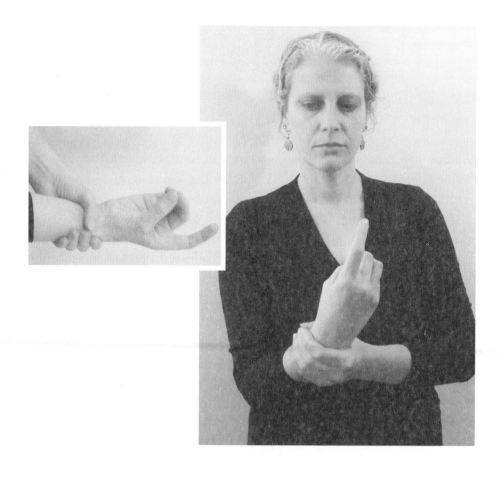

The left hand fully encircles the right wrist. The right index finger is raised and slightly bent, and it points toward the heart. The right thumb touches the closed middle, ring, and pinky fingers.

See the Forest (the Big Picture) Despite the Trees

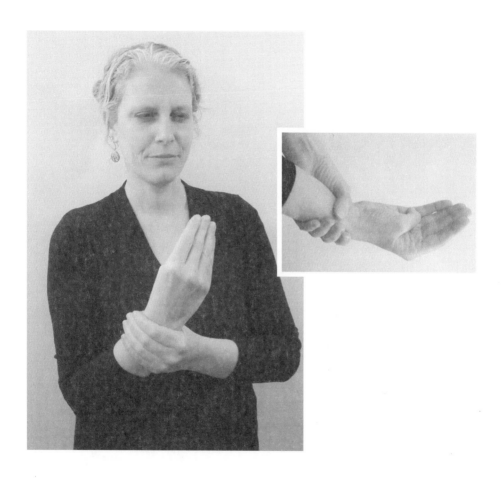

The left hand holds the right wrist. The right thumb touches the base of the right pinky finger. All the other fingers of the right hand are slightly curled and point to the heart.

Awaken
Inner Beauty

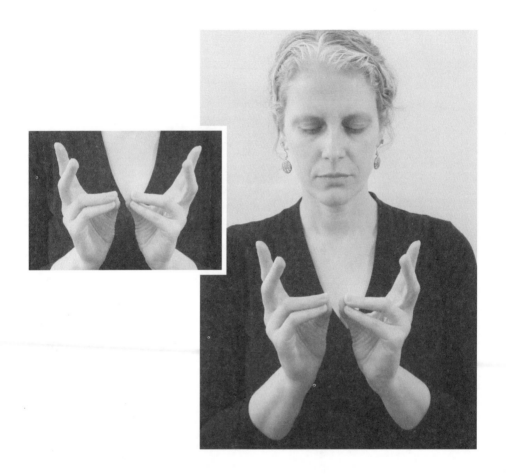

The thumb, pinky, and ring fingers of each hands are
held together. Index and middle fingers are separated.
Both hands are held in front of the heart center like a
flower opening. Breathe.

Release
Self-Sabotage

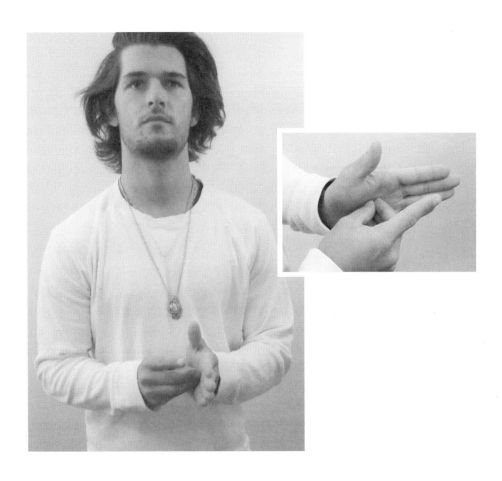

The fingers of the left hand are fully open and held in
front of the solar plexus. The right thumb touches the
middle, ring, and pinky fingers. The right index finger is
raised. The right middle, ring, and pinky fingers touch the
middle of the open left palm. Breathe. The sound that
supports this is "Amm Hoooo."

Strengthen the Heart and Mind Connection

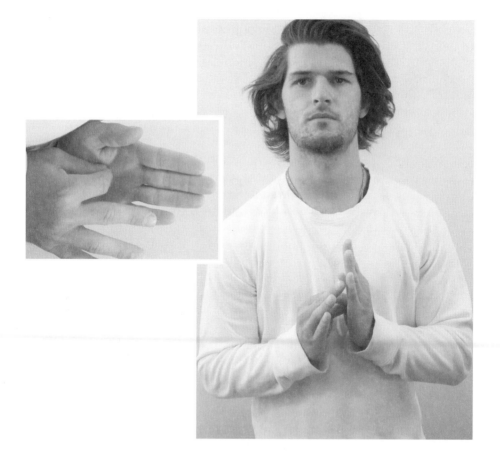

The fingers of the left hand are extended, closed, and held in front of the solar plexus. The right thumb touches the right index finger. The other fingers on the right hand are extended and open. The right thumb and index finger touch the middle of the left hand. Breathe. The sound that supports this is "Hunnnn."

Open to
Higher Communication

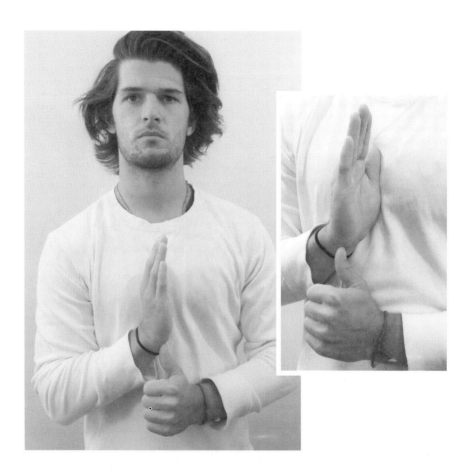

The left hand makes a fist with the thumb extended.
The fingers of the right hand are extended and closed.
The right hand is held in front of the heart. The
raised thumb of the left hand touches the bottom of
the palm of the right hand.

Find Balance and Harmony in Family Relationships

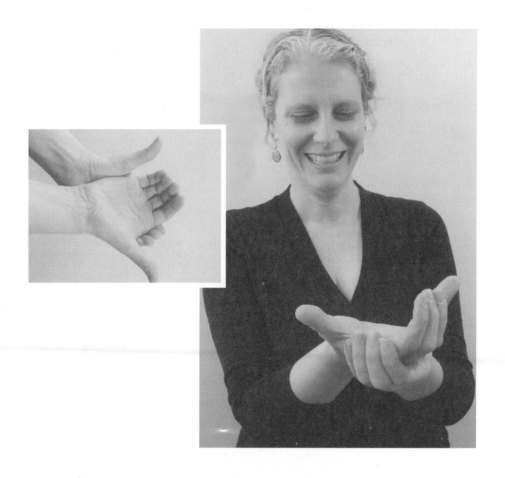

The left hand is fully open with the fingers held
together, slightly bent and cupped. The left thumb
extends outward. The right hand (palm up) rests
in the left palm, and the left hand cups the right
hand. The thumb of the right hand extends outward.

Find Harmony
with Children

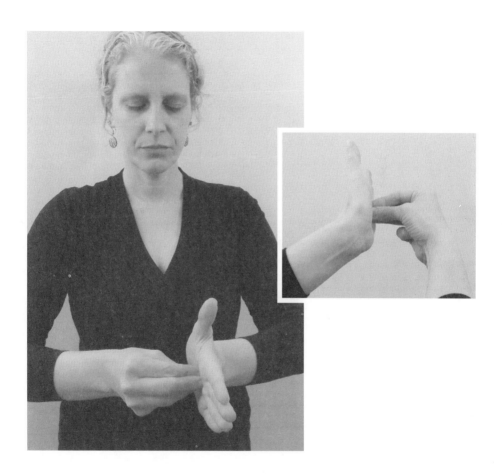

The fingers of the left hand are extended and closed.
The left hand is held in front of the middle of the
body. The right thumb touches the index, middle,
and ring fingers. The right pinky finger is closed and
touches the right palm. The fingertips of the right
hand touch the middle of the left palm.

Develop Harmony with Nature

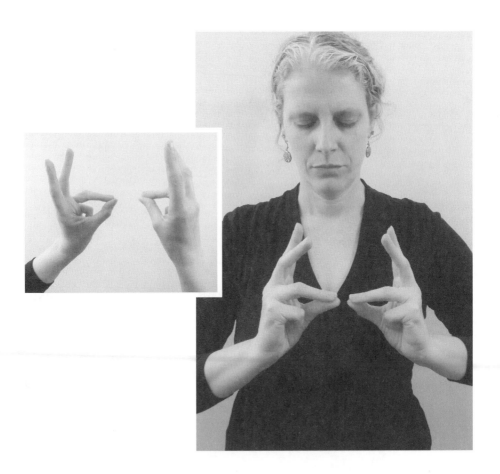

The thumbs of each hand touch the slightly bent ring fingers. The pinky fingers bend and touch the middle of the palms. Both hands are held in front of the heart. Breathe. The sound that supports this is "Asommmm."

Create Harmony with Water

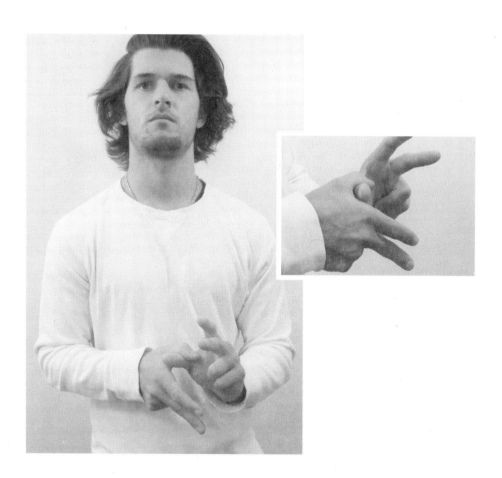

The thumbs, index fingers, and middle fingers extend and are slightly bent. The ring and pinky fingers are closed. The right thumb hooks over the left thumb, and the fingers of the right hand point downward in front of the solar plexus. Breathe. The sound that supports this is "Aaaahummmm."

Recognize Potentials, and Take Advantage of Them

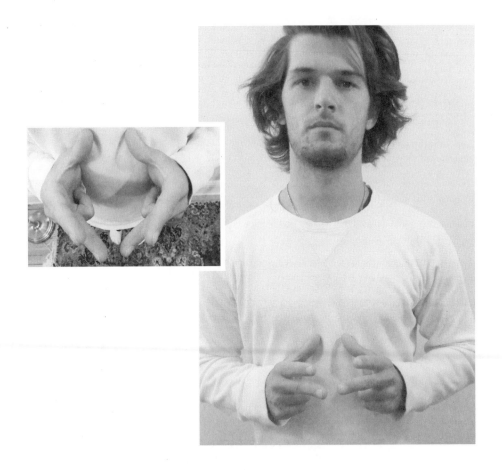

Thumbs, index, and middle fingers of both hands are extended. The ring and pinky fingers of both hands are bent and touch the middle of the palms. The extended fingers of both hands are held in front of the solar plexus. The sound that supports this is "Hummmm."

Manifest
Potentials

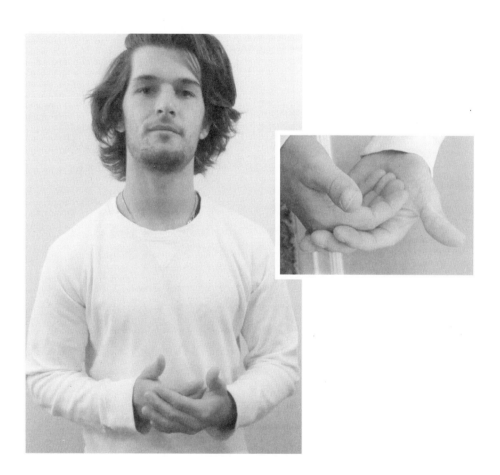

The fingers of both hands are closed, extended, and
cupped, and the thumbs point away from the cupped
fingers. The right hand (palm up) rests inside the left
hand in front of the solar plexus. Breathe. The sound
that supports this is "Manyoooo."

Summon Healing
Star Karma

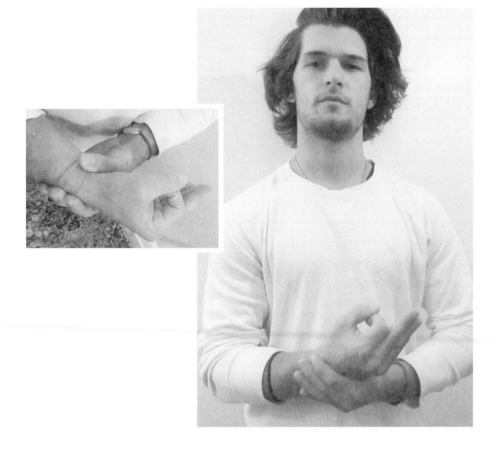

The left hand grasps the right wrist. The right thumb
rests atop the slightly bent right index finger. The
middle, ring, and pinky fingers are extended and separated, pointing toward the left side of the body near
the stomach. Breathe. The sound that supports this is
"Mayuuuoooo."

Recognize Patterns in Your Life

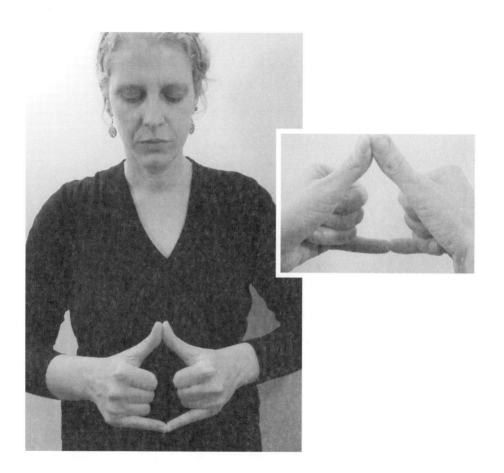

The index, middle, and ring fingers of both hands close and touch the palms. Both thumbs and pinky fingers are extended, and the tips of the thumbs and pinky fingers touch each other in front of the solar plexus. Breathe. The sound that supports this is "Anhyoooo."

Surrender to
the Situation

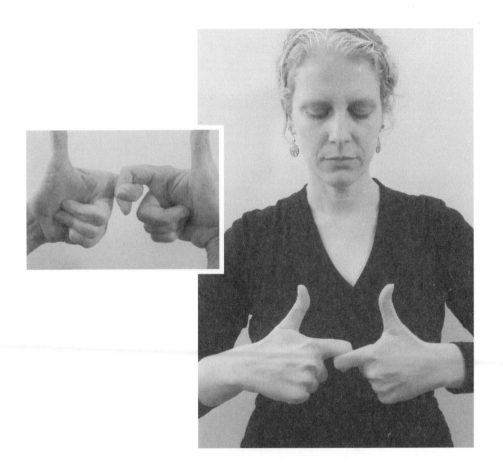

The thumbs and index fingers of both hands are
extended. The other fingers are closed and bent. The
right index finger hooks over the left index finger. This
position is held in front of the solar plexus, thumbs up.

Develop
Discretion

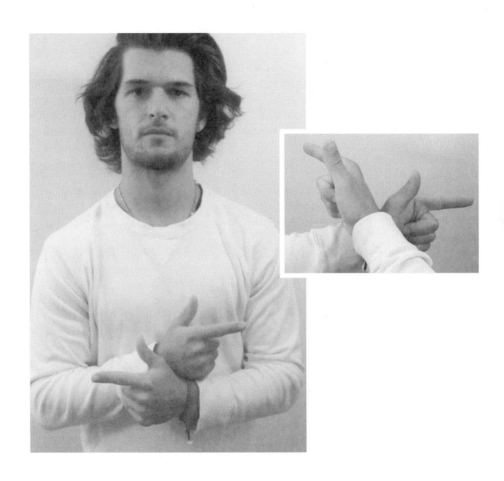

The thumbs and index fingers of both hands are
extended. The other fingers are closed and bent. Both
wrists touch, the right atop the left, and are held in
front of the heart center. Breathe.

Create
Abundance Energy

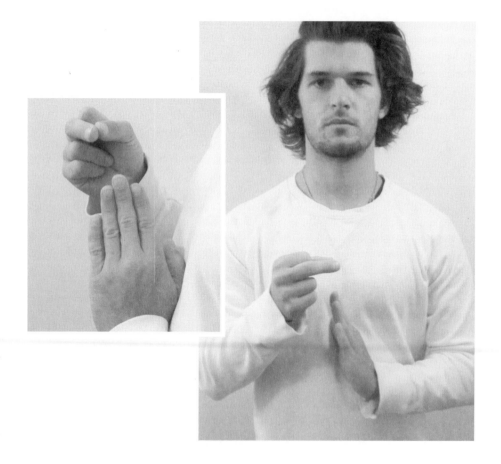

All the fingers of the left hand are extended and
closed. The left hand is held in front of the heart,
fingers pointing up. The right middle finger touches
the right thumb. The other fingers of the right hand
are closed. The right hand is held about two inches
above the left hand.

Invoke Healing
Mother Energy

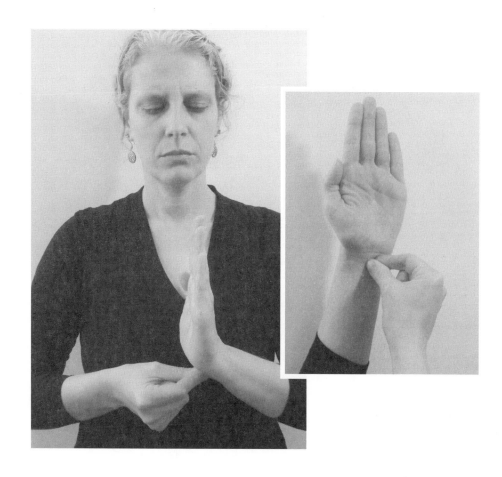

All fingers of the left hand are extended and closed,
pointing up. The right thumb touches the right index
finger and all other fingers of the right hand are
closed. The right index finger and thumb touch the
inside of the left wrist. Breathe. The sound that supports this is "Kangyo."

Request Healing
Patriarchal Energy

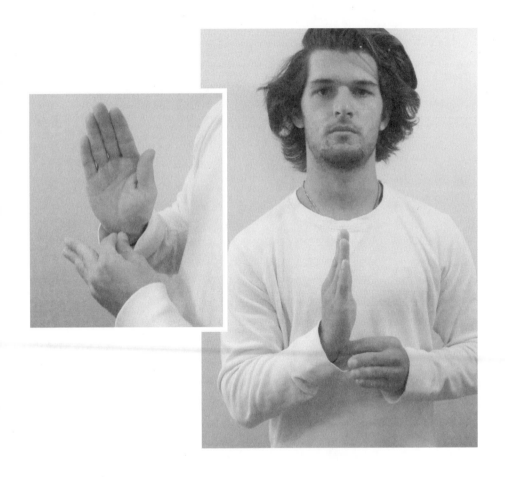

All fingers of the right hand are extended and closed,
pointing up. The left thumb touches the left index
finger and all other fingers of the left hand are closed,
extended, and point forward. The left hand touches
the inside of the right wrist.

Fully Develop
the Senses

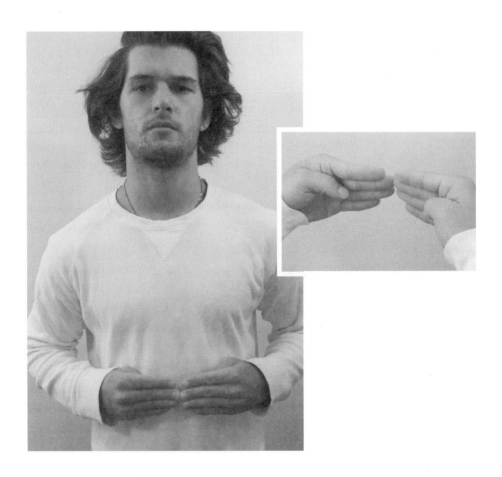

All fingers of both hands are extended and closed.
Each thumb touches its palm. Both hands are slightly
bent with fingertips touching each other. The hands
are held in front of the solar plexus.

Take Action

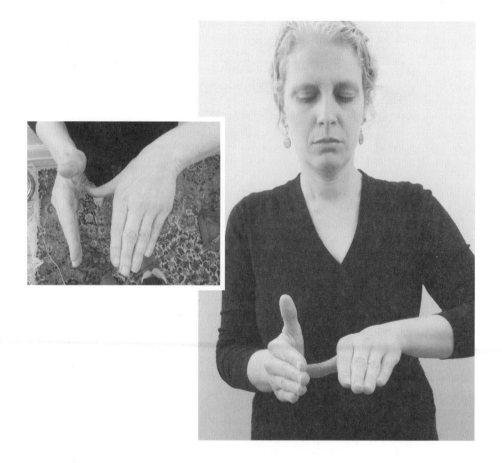

All fingers of the left hand are extended, closed, and
slightly bent and held parallel to the floor (palm
down). The left thumb is extended outward. All fingers and the thumb of the right hand are extended,
closed, and slightly bent. The extended left thumb
points to the right palm.

Create
Appreciation

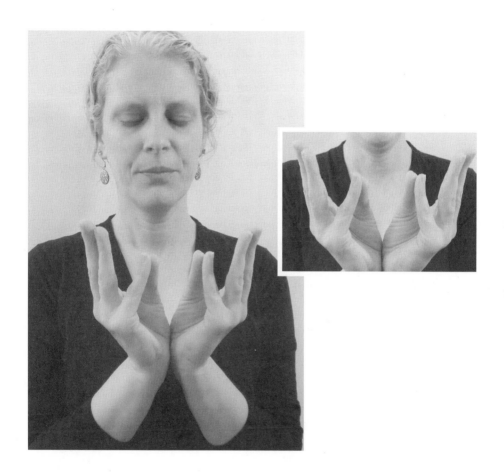

Each thumb touches the pinky fingers of its hand.
The inside of both wrists touch. The hands are held
in front of the heart center like a flower. All other fingers are closed and extended outward.

Response versus Reaction

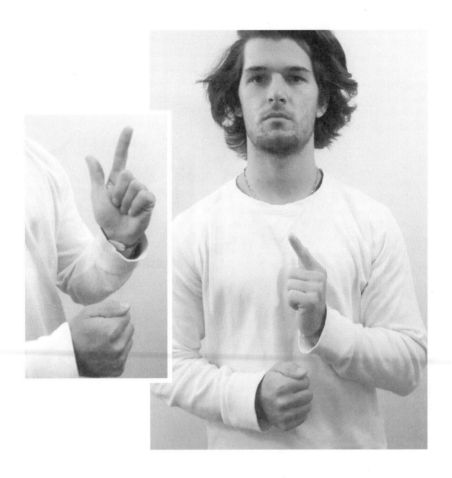

All fingers of the left hand are closed in a fist except
the index finger, which is held in front of the heart,
thumb extended. The right hand forms a fist, thumb
closed, and is held in front of the solar plexus.

Release the Fear of Dying

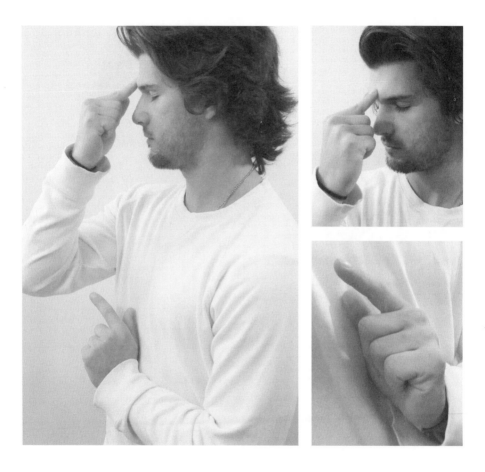

The fingers of both hands are closed in a fist except the index fingers. The extended index finger of the right hand touches the third eye. The extended index finger of the left hand is held in front of the solar plexus. Breathe. The sound that supports this is "Manfaaaarrrr."

Maintain a
Healthy Body

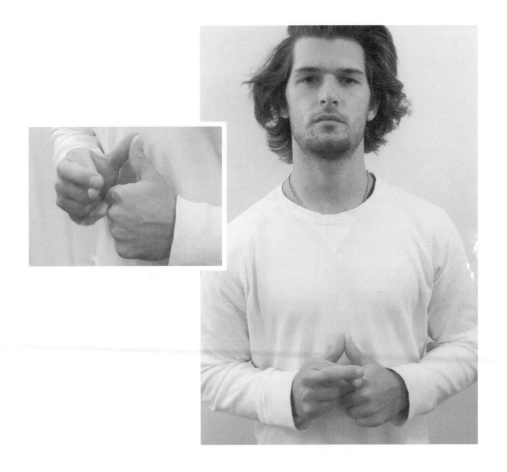

The right middle finger crosses over the right index
finger. All other fingers of the right hand are closed
in a fist. All fingers of the left hand are closed in a
fist. Extended thumbs touch to form a triangle. Both
hands are held in front of the solar plexus.

Draw Healthy Boundaries

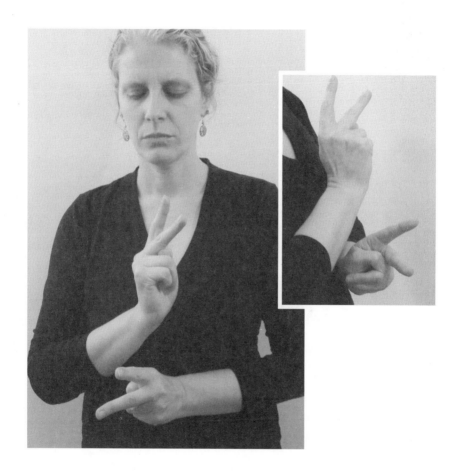

Both thumbs touch the base of both middle fingers.
Both ring and pinky fingers touch their palms.
The right hand is held in front of the heart, fingers
pointing up, and the left hand is held in front of the
solar plexus, fingers pointing forward.

Take Back
Personal Power

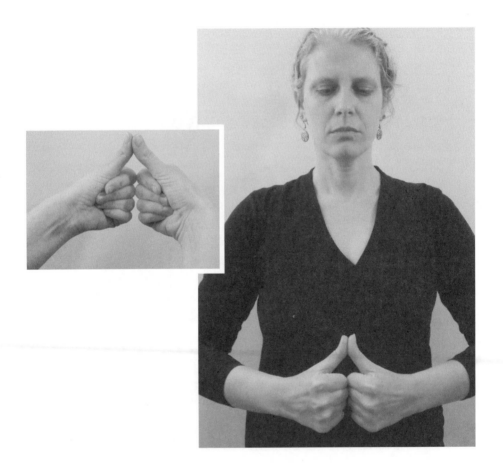

All fingers are closed in fists, and the knuckles of each
fist touch. Both extended thumbs touch. Hands are
held in front of the navel. Breathe. The sound that
supports this is "Rahaaaammmm."

Organize
Your Life

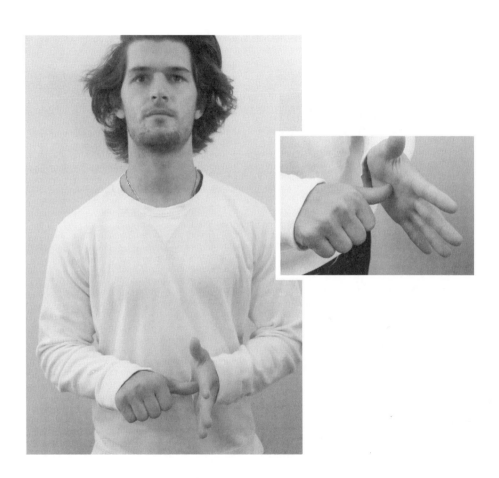

All fingers and the thumb of the left hand are open
and extended. All fingers of the right hand are closed
in a fist except the thumb. The extended right thumb
touches the middle of the left palm and is held in
front of the solar plexus.

Connect with Your Angels

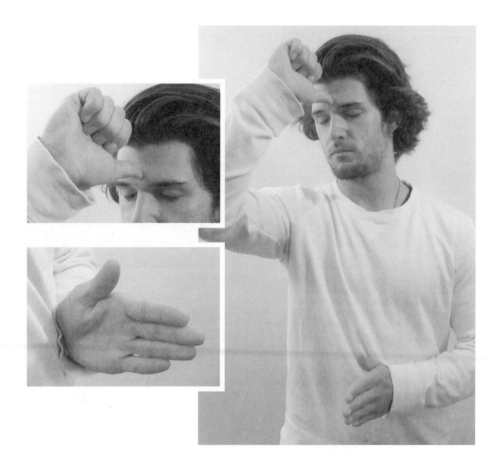

The right hand forms a fist with the thumb extended.
The right thumb touches the third eye. The fingers of
the left hand are extended and closed. The left hand
is held above your solar plexus, pointing forward.
The sound that supports this is "Ava Matta Oootttt."
Repeat this at least twenty-one times.

Request
Angel Blessings

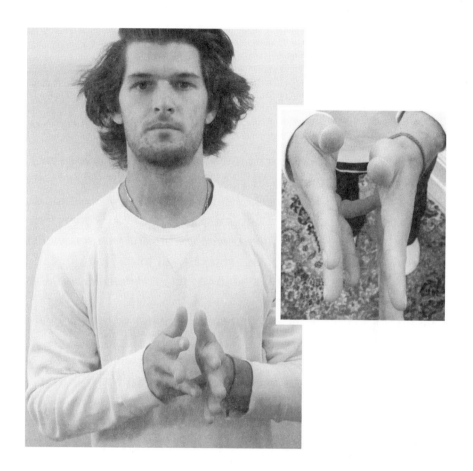

The fingers of both hands are extended and open.
The pinky finger of the right hand touches the middle
of the left palm. The thumb of the right hand is held
in front of the heart. The sound that supports this is
"Ma Kutt Oaa Iii."

Angelic Intonations to Raise Your Vibration

Archangel Michael and Angel Shamiel

Hello, my dear family, this is Archangel Michael and Angel Shamiel. The sounds listed here are from the Pleiades. The people of the Pleiades have a profound connection with angelic beings, and your DNA is from there. Some of you have had visions of Egypt that awakened your connection to ancient lands and the remembrance of who you are and why you are here.

There are some ancient chakras you can call forth. You can call for the Pleiadian chakras to be activated in the physical body. Again, this is the first time this information is coming to this world. These Pleiadian chakras are located underneath your spinal column in the back of the body, in your hip area.

All of you have star connections, for your higher selves live in twelve different realities. There are twelve chakras associated with twelve planets in the system where you exist. These chakras must be activated to have a higher reality. This way, you'll experience more of the higher reality within your physical body.

There is no wrong way of making these sounds. We ask that you make the sound with full feeling from your throat combined with the energy of your solar plexus. That is all that is needed. The key is the power of the solar plexus combined with the vocal cords.

Please note that these intonations are given in the utmost sacredness. When these sounds are practiced with sacredness and the deepest gratitude from your heart, you will create miracles. You will create fire within you, the energy that can liberate human beings.

When you make these intonations, you might feel energy in the top of your head. It might feel like a mild burning sensation. Do these gently, for you could feel spaced out from the energy. Making these sounds can liberate you very quickly.

"Ka Att Maido"
(I am peaceful. I have angelic peace.)

"Eaha Va Pine"
(I am graceful.)

"Mane Lii Ho"
(I am clear in my life.)

"Mahido Mahadevate"
(I know.)

"Suran Ho"
(I have angelic power.)

"Sa Him Ka Laii"
(I am.)

"Van Muda Van Ha"
(I am one with the angelic presence.)

"Van Ha Van Sa Van Bi"
(My path is open.)

"Kaha Shi Kaho Modo"
(My angels light my path.)

"Maho Siomm"
(Angels are my guiding light.)

"Samhe Von Mayuon"
(I call on the angel of strength and power.)

"Arhan Go"
(I call on earth angels to balance me.)

"H Yuon Hyo"
(My power comes from the angels.)

"Maa Oott Maa Mmm"
(I ask for angelic love.)

"Gumm Si Rehmo"
(I ask for angelic discretion.)

"Sar Dor Lahim"
(I am an individual, but I also belong to the group.)

"Lee Aaavv Ro"
(I take action.)

"Sardi Dharum"
(Heaven and earth are balanced in my life.)

"Kinshi Mo Haido"
(I awaken to my star connection and my star heritage.)

"Ooammmm Lo Ward"
(My path is clear.)

"Kim Maido Ka La Wata"
(God is my goal.)

"Arham Lave"
(I am the creative force.)

"Manbhi Ka Ra Wata"
(I am complete and whole.)

"Singme Wanchi Li"
(I awaken the goddess within me.)

"Sanho Makai Huaee Ummm"
(I integrate my soul, monad, and I Am presence.)

"Mailo Manuaa Seehom"
(I integrate the twelve aspects of my I Am presence.)

"Citrimm Rave To"
(My inner child is healed and happy.)

"Aaramsu Aaarihane"
(I am worthy and deserving.)

"Kunaal Lahom Paa"
(I am becoming expansive.)

"Anngi Andon Hinge"
(I heal my birth trauma.)

"Karas Ka Loi Zing Wa"
(I am becoming my natural self.)

"Wase Sarito Liam"
(My karma with all animals is healed.)

"Kum Cegot Kingla Maria"
(I heal my family lineage karma.)

"Sari Do Wa Maee"
(I break all the promises made to God to remain poor,
single, ill, and in bondage.)

"Kari Kari Si Hoto"
(I am my own master.)

"Xant Labda So La Ee"
(I break group karma, such as cult, military ties, or group mentality.)

"Va Len Vas So"
(I Heal the fear and let go.)

"Larun Maiwa Li Eehmm"
(I am in the flow of life.)

"Osammm Sahe Lahm"
(I heal family unit karma.)

"Rikosmm Rahml Risolomm"
(I accept and love my physical body.)

Breathing Exercises to Integrate Celestial Energy

Archangel Michael

To do these breathing exercises, observe your body while you breathe. Feel your power change as you breathe. When you have agitated thoughts, your breathing will shift the energies. Try to do this breathing in a controlled way so that an equal amount of breath goes in and out. By simply observing your body, you will be able to regulate your breathing to do these exercises.

🌸 To make fast, strong connections with the angelic kingdom, breathe in through both the ears and out through the forehead.

🌸 To release stress and tension, breathe in blue, pink, and white through the crown chakra and out through the mouth.

🌸 To activate the ascension chakra, breathe in through the eyebrows and out through the medulla oblongata.

🌸 To feel power and courage, breathe in through both closed fists and out through the crown chakra.

🌸 Open a portal to star systems and galaxies by breathing in through the bottom of the eyes and releasing through the crown chakra.

🌸 Open to higher truths and perception by breathing evenly through both nostrils while pressing two fingers of each hand on both eyebrows.

🌸 Become flexible and open by breathing through the openings of the fully opened fingers of both hands.

❧ To make the heart strong, make a fist with the left hand, and place it on top of the right side of the heart while breathing normally through both nostrils.

❧ To feel grounded and reassured, breathe through the toes, and release through the toes.

❧ To disconnect from Earth gravity, breathe through the front of the toes and release through the backs of the ankles. (This will help you accept newer and higher truths, and not become caught in rigid ideas. This is also the first step in levitation and is best practiced for fifteen minutes each day.)

❧ To feel energized and vibrant, breathe in through the tongue, and release through the ears.

❧ Take action by breathing in through the hair (on the head) and releasing through the fingernails.

❧ To release karmic energy related to life patterns, breathe in through the eyes, and release through both shoulders.

❧ Dissolve escapist energy by breathing in through the naval and releasing through the legs. This can support your commitment to finish all you have come here to complete.

❧ To balance your male and female energy, breathe in through the left side of the neck and release through the right side of the body and vice versa.

❧ Know your life path by breathing in through the forehead and releasing through the toes.

❧ Open the mahatma energy and activate the platinum ray by breathing in through the thymus [near the heart] and releasing through the back of the hands. (This is only for advanced and serious spiritual students.)

❧ Coordinate graceful body movements by breathing in through the fully opened right palm onto the fully opened left palm.

❧ To remember your sacred divinity, make a circle using the thumb and index finger of your right hand. Breathe in through the circle, take the breath through the nose, and exhale through the legs.

❀ Open vertical and horizontal wisdom by holding your fully opened right hand straight in front of your solar plexus. The opened left hand is held straight in front of your heart chakra. Breathe in through both nostrils.

❀ To ground the energy of what you intend to create, the right open palm faces upward, and the left open palm faces downward. Breathe in through both nostrils.

❀ Feel courageous and confident by forming fists of both the hands. Bring the right fist on top of the left fist, and breathe.

❀ To feel secure in your life, close all fingers, and raise your thumbs. Bring both hands in front of your heart, and breathe.

❀ To identify your priorities, make fists with both hands, and bring them in front of your solar plexus, pointing downward. Breathe in through both nostrils consistently. (This will help bring you back to yourself.)

❀ If you become lost in others, fully open the left hand, and place it on the solar plexus, touching the naval. The right index and the middle fingers are open and face outward. (This can bring you back to yourself.)

❀ To balance the energies of the spirit and material worlds, make circles with the thumb and index fingers of both hands. Bring your hands between your heart and solar plexus chakras. Breathe consistently through both the nostrils.

About Rae Chandran

Rae Chandran was born in India and has lived in the United States and Japan. He performs individual channeling sessions for his clients, and his articles have been published in the *Sedona Journal of Emergence!* Rae teaches workshops throughout the Far East on the Ancient Egyptian mysteries, DNA activation, and channeling. He creates soul symbols for his clients, and he leads tours of ancient holy places worldwide.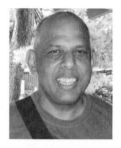

Rae founded the Omran Institute, which promotes DNA awareness and certifies practitioners of Omran 12-Strand DNA Activation. He also performs individual Omran 12-Strand DNA sessions for his clients. Rae lives with his wife and children outside of Tokyo, Japan. Form more information, visit his website at www.RaeChandran.com.

About Robert Mason Pollock

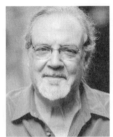

Robert Mason Pollock was born in Washington, DC, and has lived in London (England), Canada, and the Berkshire mountains of Massachusetts. He is an energy healer at a holistic health resort in the Berkshires, and he has an energy healing practice with locations in New York City and the Berkshires.

Robert wrote *Navigating by Heart*. He teaches workshops in spirituality and DNA activation. He also performs individual Omran 12-Strand DNA sessions for his clients. Robert currently lives in the Berkshires. For more information, visit his website at www.BerkshireEnergyHealing.com.

THROUGH RAE CHANDRAN

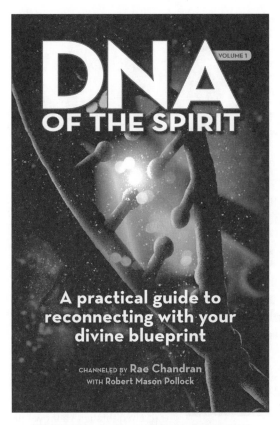

$19.95 • Softcover • 384 pp. • ISBN: 978-1-62233-013-3

32 color pages of mudras and images
to activate your 12 levels of DNA

DNA of the Spirit, Volume 1

The etheric strands of your DNA are the information library of your soul. They contain the complete history of you, lifetime after lifetime; a record of the attitudes, karma, and emotional predispositions you brought into this lifetime; and a blueprint, or lesson plan, for your self-improvement. Your DNA is also a record of your existence from the moment of your creation as a starbeing to your present incarnation. This information is written in every cell of your body.

CHAPTERS INCLUDE

- Mudras for Activating the Twelve Layers of DNA
- The Awakening of Crystalline Consciousness
- Auspicious Times for Awakening Consciousness
- Angelic Support for DNA Activation
- The History of Human DNA
- Your Internal Compass: Nature's Body Intelligence

THROUGH RAE CHANDRAN

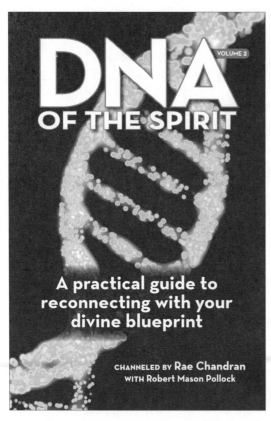

$16.95 • Softcover • 192 pp. • 978-1-62233-027-0

DNA of the Spirit, Volume 2

This companion book to *DNA of the Spirit, Volume 1* originated with the intention and desire to bring forth understanding to support humanity. Go through this volume while holding a sacredness inside of you, asking that the material be imprinted in your sacredness so that it may become an experience that you will be able to live.

Some of the material in this book is coded, and sincere students will find they can open these codes. Understanding can be received through your own filter and in your own way. This way, you will find the Divine within.

CHAPTERS INCLUDE

- Auric Imprinting Technique for Healing
- The Number of God
- Reveal Your Life Contracts
- Re-create Your Life with Your Akashic Records

- Humans Are Creators in Training
- Use Shape-Shifting for Regeneration
- How to Activate the Codes Within You
- From Darkness unto Light: the Aquarian Age

- Discover Your Energy Connections to Beings of Light
- Understand the Sacred Geometry of the Human Body
- Determine What Drives Your Soul

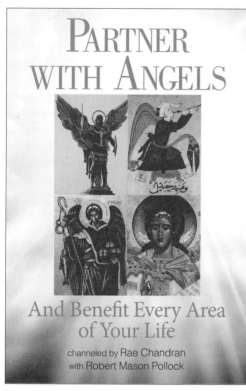

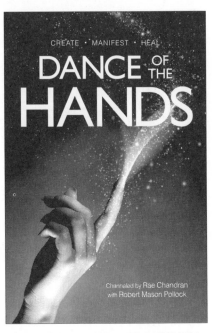
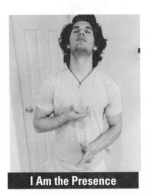
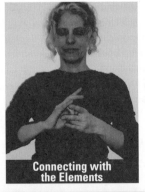
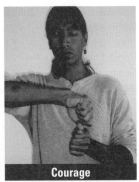

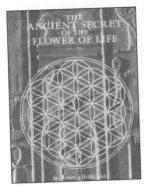
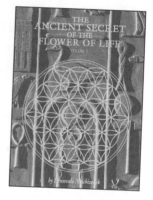
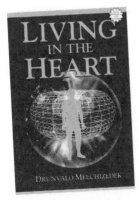
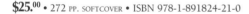

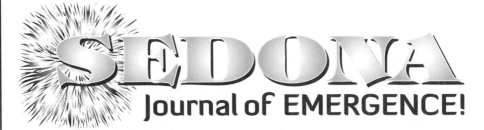
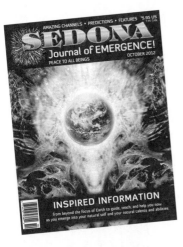

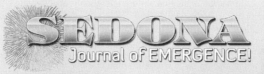
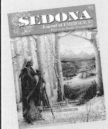
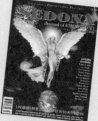

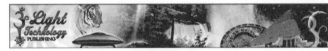
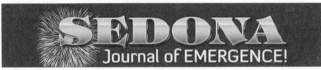
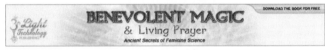
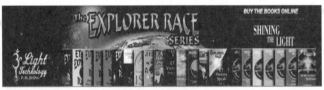
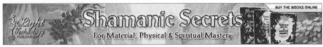